VASCULAR DISEASE
A HANDBOOK FOR NURSES

A Practical approach for Medical and Nursing Staff, offers a step-by-step guide to caring for patients in a variety of clinical settings. It follows a patient's path of care from management in the outpatient clinic, through to the hospital ward, theatre, recovery room and back to the follow-up outpatient clinic. A clear, concise format is used throughout the book, with reference to evidence-based interventions and the physiology underpinning them, and the use of simple line diagrams and treatment flow charts to illustrate the essential aspects of care.

Edited by a vascular nurse and a vascular surgeon, with contributions from a group of invited authors, the book reflects the multidisciplinary nature of patient care and will be a valuable resource for nurses, surgeons and other healthcare professionals involved in caring for this patient group.

VASCULAR DISEASE

A HANDBOOK FOR NURSES

Haytham Al-Khaffaf
Consultant Vascular Surgeon, Vascular Unit,
Burnley General Hospital

Sharon Dorgan
Vascular Nurse Consultant
Burnley Healthcare NHS Trust
Casterton Avenue
Burnley Lancs BB10 2PQ

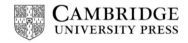

CAMBRIDGE
UNIVERSITY PRESS

PUBLISHED BY THE PRESS SYNDICATE OF THE UNIVERSITY OF CAMBRIDGE
The Pitt Building, Trumpington Street, Cambridge, United Kingdom

CAMBRIDGE UNIVERSITY PRESS
The Edinburgh Building, Cambridge CB2 2RU, UK
40 West 20th Street, New York, NY 10011-4211, USA
477 Williamstown Road, Port Melbourne, VIC 3207, Australia
Ruiz de Alarcón 13, 28014 Madrid, Spain
Dock House, The Waterfront, Cape Town 8001, South Africa

http://www.cambridge.org

First published 2005

Printed in the United Kingdom at the University Press, Cambridge

Typeface: Minion 11/12.5pt   System: QuarkXpress®

A catalogue record for this book is available from the British Library

ISBN 0 521 67451 4

The publisher has used its best endeavours to ensure that the URLs
for external websites referred to in this book are correct and
active at the time of going to press. However, the publisher has
no responsibility for the websites and can make no guarantee
that a site will remain live or that the content is or will
remain appropriate.

Every effort has been made in preparing this book to provide accurate and
up-to-date information that is in accord with accepted standards and
practice at the time of publication. Nevertheless, the authors, editors and
publisher can make no warranties that the information contained herein is
totally free from error, not least because clinical standards are constantly
changing through research and regulation. The authors, editors and
publisher therefore disclaim all liability for direct or consequential
damages resulting from the use of material contained in this book. Readers
are strongly advised to pay careful attention to information provided by
the manufacturer of any drugs or equipment that they plan to use.

CONTENTS

LIST OF ABBREVIATIONS

AAA	Abdominal aortic aneurysm
ABPI	Ankle brachial pressure index
AF	Atrial fibrillation
AIE	Acute inflammatory episode
ASA	American Society of Anaesthesiologists
ATLS	Advanced trauma life support
AVPU	Alert, verbal, painful, unresponsive
BP	Blood pressure
CCU	Critical care unit
CHD	Coronary heart disease
CMI	Chronic mesenteric ischaemia
CNS	Clinical nurse specialist
COPD	Chronic obstructive pulmonary disease
CPAP	Continuous positive airway pressure
CSF	Cerebrospinal fluid
CT	Computerised tomography
CVA	Cerebrovascular accident
CVP	Central venous pressure
CXR	Chest X-ray
DGH	District general hospital
DHSS	Department of Health and Social Security
DNA	Deoxyribo nucleic acid
DoH	Department of Health
DP	Dorsalis pedis
DSC	Disablement services centre
DVT	Deep venous thrombosis
ECG	Electrocardiograph
ePTFE	Expanded poly tetra fluoro ethylene
ESR	Erythrocyte sedimentation rate
ETS	Endoscopic thoracic sympathectomy
EVAR	Endo-vascular aortic aneurysm repair
FBC	Full blood count
FFP	Fresh frozen plasma
GA	General anaesthesia

GCS	Glasgow coma scale
GP	General practitioner
HRT	Hormone replacement therapy
I/V	Inspiration/ventilation
ICP	Integrated care pathways
IHD	Ischemic heart disease
IPOP	Immediate post-operative protheses
IPPV	Invasive positive pressure ventilation
ITU	Intensive therapy unit
LDL	Low density lipoprotein
LLI	Lower limb ischaemia
LMWH	Low molecular weight heparin
MASS	Multi-centre aneurysm screening study
MDT	Multi-disciplinary team
MI	Myocardial infarction
MLD	Manual lymphatic drainage
MLLB	Multi-layer lymphoedema bandaging
MMPs	Matrix metalloproteinase proteinases
MRA	Magnetic resonance arteriography
MRI	Magnetic resonance imaging
NHS	National Health Service
NIPPV	Non-invasive positive pressure ventilation
OPD	Outpatient Department
PAD	Peripheral arterial disease
PAFC	Pulmonary artery flotation catheter
PAM	Post-amputation mobility
PAWP	Pulmonary artery wedge pressure
PCA	Patient-controlled analgesia
PEG	Percutaneous endoscopic gastronomy
PT	Posterior tibial
PTB	Patella tendon bearing
PVD	Peripheral vascular disease
RA	Regional anaesthesia
RP	Raynaud's phenomenon
RTA	Road traffic accident
SLD	Simple lymphatic drainage
SSS	Subclavian steal syndrome
TIA	Transient ischaemic attack
TIVA	Total intravenous anaesthesia
TOS	Thoracic outlet syndrome
t-PA	Tissue plasminogen activator
TC	Total serum cholesterol
U/E	Urea and electrolytes
U&E	Urea and electrolytes
US	Ultrasound
VAS	Visual analogue scales

LIST OF CONTRIBUTORS

Haytham Al-Khaffaf
Consultant Vascular Surgeon
Vascular Unit
Burnley General Hospital

Julie Bells
Theatre Sister
Burnley General Hospital

Francis J. Boon
Consultant in Rehabilitation
    Medicine
Preston Disablement Centre
Royal Preston Hospital

Sharon Dorgan
Vascular Nurse Consultant
Vascular Unit
Burnley General Hospital

Omer Ehsan
Senior House Officer
Vascular Unit
Burnley General Hospital

Marcia Gore
Tissue Viability Nurse
East Lancashire Hospitals NHS Trust

Susan Greenwood
Pain Specialist Nurse
Burnley General Hospital

Susan Jane
Practice Development Facilitator
Burnley General Hospital

Kath Payton
Leg Ulcer Nurse
Burnley
Pendle and Rossendale Primary
Care Trust

Asad Rahi
Consultant Vascular Surgeon
Vascular Unit
Burnley General Hospital

Ferdinand Serracino-Inglott
Specialist Registrar
Vascular Unit
Burnley General Hospital

Ayad Shakir
Consultant Anaesthetist
Burnley General Hospital

Valerie Skinner
Clinical Effectiveness Manager
East Lancashire Hospitals NHS Trust

Christine Spencer
Vascular Technologist
Vascular Unit
Burnley General Hospital

William Stevenson
Consultant Radiologist
X-Ray Department
Burnley General Hospital

Lynda Thompson
Vascular Nurse Specialist
Burnley General Hospital
East Lancashire Hospitals NHS Trust

James C. Watts
Consultant in Anaesthesia and
    Intensive Care
East Lancashire Trust

Michelle Weddell
Diabetic Podiatrist
East Lancashire Trust

Justine Whitaker
Macmillan Lymphoedema Clinical
    Specialist
East Lancashire Hospice
Blackburn
Lancashire

PREFACE

The management of patients with vascular disease is complex and requires a multi-disciplinary approach of which nurses play an integral part. Recent years have witnessed the development of vascular nursing in the UK as a specialist area, with appointments of vascular nurse specialists and nurse consultants.

Specialist vascular courses are now available for nurses in the UK and vascular nurses have their own professional society.

This book aims to provide nurses with the appropriate knowledge to meet the challenge of caring for patients with vascular disease. It is designed to be an easy to use guide and not as an exhaustive textbook. Additional sources will need to be accessed to provide any further required information.

The book is separated into parts in accordance to patients potential journey from outpatient department or emergency admission, through to investigations, nursing care on the ward, surgical and radiological intervention, intensive care unit (ICU) or high-dependency unit (HDU), rehabilitation to discharge back into the community.

This approach has been chosen to show the complex inter-twinning of departments and staff involved in caring for this patient group. Each chapter will also address the role of the nurse in a specific area of care.

Charts, diagrams and pictures have been used to highlight important points and make the book an easy read. A reference list has also been provided at the end of each chapter.

Finally we would like to thank all the authors who have contributed to this book. We would also like to thank Madiha Rafi for her help with the artwork.

Haytham Al-Khaffaf
Consultant Vascular Surgeon

Sharon Dorgan
Vascular Nurse Consultant

OUTPATIENT DEPARTMENT

This chapter outlines the main arterial and venous diseases that are likely to be seen within a vascular outpatient setting. It also highlights the role of the vascular nurse specialist wherever appropriate.

1.1   Peripheral arterial disease
        S. Dorgan and H. Al-Khaffaf

1.2   Carotid artery disease
        S. Dorgan and H. Al-Khaffaf

1.3   Abdominal aortic aneurysm
        S. Dorgan and H. Al-Khaffaf

1.4   Upper limb ischaemia
        H. Al-Khaffaf

1.5   Raynaud's phenomenon
        S. Dorgan

1.6   Vasculitis
        S. Dorgan and H. Al-Khaffaf

1.7   Thoracic outlet syndrome
        S. Dorgan

1.8   Hyperhydrosis
        S. Dorgan and H. Al-Khaffaf

1.1   PERIPHERAL ARTERIAL DISEASE

S. Dorgan and H. Al-Khaffaf

Peripheral arterial disease (PAD) is generally used to describe diseases of the arteries outside the heart and the brain. However, specifically it refers to atherosclerosis of the arteries that carry blood to the legs (and to a lesser extent to the arms).

ATHEROSCLEROSIS

Atherosclerosis is a complex and insidious condition, and one of the primary causes of death in the UK.

Generally, arteries have smooth linings, allowing unimpaired blood flow. Atherosclerosis is a degenerative arterial disease and refers to "hardening of the arteries", whereby muscle and elastic tissues are replaced with fibrous tissue, and calcification might occur.

It is characterised by atheromatous plaques, which are deposits of fatty material in the lining of medium- and large-sized arteries. These arteries then become narrowed and rough as more fat is deposited. Blood clots form more easily due to their roughness, further narrowing the artery, and thus potentially limiting blood flow.

A reduction of blood supply to the organs and tissues means that they are unable to perform as well, and the plaques are very liable to break down and form ulcers. Thromboses may then develop as a result of the roughening and ulceration of the inner coat of the arteries (Figure 1.1.1).

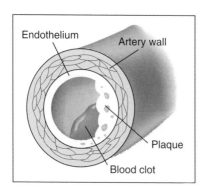

Fig. 1.1.1: A cross section of a diseased artery.

Table 1.1.1: Areas of the body that are affected by atherosclerosis

Affected area	Disease type	Clinical effects
Brain	Cerebral vascular disease	TIA/amaurosis fugax/CVA
Heart	Coronary artery disease	Myocardial infarction
		Angina
Abdomen	Aortic artery disease	Aortic aneurysm
Renal	Renal artery disease	Renal failure
		Hypertension
Lower limbs	Peripheral arterial disease	Intermittent claudication
		Chronic limb ischaemia
		Acute limb ischaemia

Signs and symptoms

Atherosclerosis causes:

- The narrowing of small arteries which reduces the blood supply to various organs and tissues.
- Occlusion as a result of thrombosis which occurs in the diseased arteries.

In many arteries, atherosclerosis might have little effect, however, in certain organs it does produce well-recognised diseases.

- In the leg arteries results in intermittent claudication and peripheral thrombosis with gangrene of the limb.
- In the cerebral arteries it leads to cerebral thrombosis (one form of "stroke").
- In the coronary arteries it leads to angina pectoris and coronary thrombosis.
- In the kidneys it causes renal artery stenosis, which may lead to hypertension and renal failure (Table 1.1.1).

CARDIOVASCULAR RISK FACTORS

PAD risk factors are those factors that are statistically associated with the incidence of the disease. The probability of developing PAD, coronary heart disease (CHD) or cerebrovascular disease is mainly dependent on a person's risk profile. PAD usually co-exists with extensive atherosclerotic disease elsewhere and, therefore, the risk of all types of vascular events for these patients is extremely high (Mikhaildis, 2000). Therefore, patients presenting with intermittent claudication require a critical assessment of all the vascular risk factors (Table 1.1.2), with the aim of reducing coronary and cerebral events risk (Belch, 1999).

Table 1.1.2: Cardiovascular risk factors for PAD

Modifiable risk factors	Non-modifiable risk factors
• Cigarette smoking • Hypercholesterolaemia • Hypertension • Physical inactivity • Obesity • Diabetes mellitus • Homocysteine (raised levels) • Thrombogenic factors	• Age • Gender • Family history

Ref.: Pasternak *et al.*, 1996.

Evidence of the benefit of correction of associated risk factors is strong (Hiatt, 2001). Conservative treatment centres on modifying the following risk factors:

- smoking cigarettes (Levy, 1989);
- hypertension (Strano *et al.*, 1993);
- diabetes mellitus (Beks *et al.*, 1995);
- hyperlipidaemia (Fowkes *et al.*, 1995);
- thrombotic abnormalities, such as platelet aggregation (Belch *et al.*, 1984), increased plasma fibrinogen (Lowe *et al.*, 1991) and decreased fibrinolysis (Smith *et al.*, 1993).

Cigarette smoking

Some 90% of PAD patients are smokers or recent ex-smokers (Mikhailidis, 2000).

Smoking is a major risk factor in lower limb atherosclerosis progression and moderate cigarette smoking (15 cigarettes a day) almost doubles the risk of developing PAD, as compared to non-smokers, and the risk may increase in relation to the number of cigarettes smoked (Hughson *et al.*, 1978; Kannel & McGee, 1985).

Studies show a four- to nine-fold increased risk of PAD in patients smoking in excess of 20 cigarettes per day, as compared to non-smokers (Hughson *et al.*, 1978).

As smoking tobacco increases the risk of intermittent claudication and contributes to its progression (Krupski, 1991), stopping smoking could prevent patients from progressing towards critical limb ischaemia and is probably the most important action a claudicant can take.

Hypertension

Hypertension increases the incidence of PAD by 4 times in women and 2.5 times in men (Kannell & McGee, 1985).

Guidelines issued by the British Hypertension Society (1999) recommend that therapy should be commenced in all patients with sustained systolic blood pressure >160 mmHg or sustained diastolic blood pressures >100 mmHg. Where there is evidence of cardiovascular disease (to include intermittent claudication), drug therapy should be initiated when patients have sustained systolic blood pressures between 140 and 159 mmHg or diastolic blood pressures between 90 and 99 mmHg.

In addition to patients commencing on any required antihypertensive medications, lifestyle modification should also be emphasised which includes:

- reduce salt intake,
- decrease alcohol consumption,
- weight reduction,
- increase exercise.

Diabetes

PAD is present in some 40% of diabetic patients aged over 40 years, and its prevalence is 7 times greater in non-insulin-dependent diabetic patients than in non-diabetics: 22% versus 3% (Beach *et al.*, 1988).

The exact nature of how diabetes increases risk of atherosclerosis is not known, however, Colwell (1987) suggests it may be due to the endothelial damage caused by free fatty acids, hyperlipidaemia, hyperglycaemia and glucose metabolism.

Levels of low- and very-low-density lipoprotein (LDL) cholesterol are often raised in people with diabetes, both of which enhance plaque formation. Conversely, high-density lipoprotein cholesterol, considered to protect against atherosclerosis, is reduced by diabetes.

Approximately 50% of all patients with diabetes will have evidence of PAD 10–15 years after the onset of diabetes. It is important for all patients with diabetes to have good diabetic control, but perhaps this is even more important in those with any form of established vascular disease.

Hyperlipidaemia

Raised serum total cholesterol, low serum high-density lipoprotein cholesterol and raised serum triglycerides are recognised risk factors that lead to PAD.

Raised lipid levels can lead to early vascular damage (fatty streaks), cholesterol rich plaques can occlude and narrow vessels, and finally endothelial function is disturbed which affects flow in the microcirculation (Belch *et al.*, 1984).

Therefore, lowering plasma lipid levels with drugs such as statins benefits patients at risk of cardiovascular events.

The current recommendation of treating only total cholesterol over 5 mmol/l has been challenged by evidence that statins may have a direct beneficial effect on atherosclerosis (Shearman, 2002). Results from studies currently underway are needed to evaluate this in greater detail, in particular the cost-effectiveness of more widespread use of these drugs (Leng *et al.*, 2001).

Antiplatelet medication

Patients with established atheromatous vascular disease are advised to take 75 mg aspirin daily, which significantly reduces cardiovascular events – 27% relative risk reduction (Antiplatelet Trialists' Collaboration, 1988).

A randomised clinical trial comparing clopidogrel (an antiplatelet agent) with aspirin (CAPRIE Trial) illustrated a significant reduction in anticipated cardiovascular events, with clopidogrel fairing slightly better (relative risk reduction of 9%). The subgroup with PAD appeared to benefit most and there appears little doubt that all claudicants should be on an appropriate antiplatelet agent (CAPRIE Steering Committee, 1996).

Gender and age

Previous studies also indicate that 2–3 times more middle-aged men than women suffer from PAD, a ratio which appears to even out over the age of 70 years (Kannel & McGee, 1985).

Approximately 20% of men over the age of 50 years are affected (Schroll & Munck, 1981). Prevalence increases with age and the condition is likely to become increasingly common as the proportion of elderly people in the population increases (Kannel, 1996).

Role of nurses in the management of cardiovascular risk factors

- *Smoking*: Advise on how smoking affects the circulation. Refer to local specialist smoking cessation service. Give constant support and encouragement to help patient quit.

- *Cholesterol*: Ensure patient has had fasting lipid profile undertaken in the last 12 months and that total serum cholesterol (TC) levels are <5 mmol/l and LDL <3 mmol/l. If above these levels request for patient to be commenced on statin (cholesterol lowering medication – for life) and advise regarding low-fat diet.
- *Hypertension*: Target levels – no diabetes <140/85 mmHg; diabetes <140/80 mmHg.
- *Antiplatelet medication*: Aspirin 75 mg once daily if no contraindications. Clopidogrel (Plavix) 75 mg once daily if unable to tolerate aspirin.
- *Exercise*: Refer to local community sports centre or hospital-based exercise programme if available. Home exercise programme should be discussed if preferred or if no other suitable alternative.
- *Diabetes*: Test patients for undiagnosed diabetes by undertaking fasting glucose test and urinalysis. Abnormal results should be passed onto the Diabetes Care Team for further assessment and management.

CHRONIC LOWER LIMB ISCHAEMIA

Chronic lower limb ischaemia (LLI) is one of the most common referrals to a vascular outpatient clinic. It becomes increasingly common with age and approximately 5% of people over 50 years have LLI. It is more common in men with a ratio of males to females of 2:1.

Symptoms

- Many patients with LLI have no symptoms.
- Only less than half of these patients typically experience cramp-like pain of the leg muscles, which is known as *intermittent claudication* (derived from the Latin word claudicatio, to limp).
- Typically the pain is brought on by exercise and relieved by rest.
- The pain only affects the muscle group being exercised: claudication involving the calf muscles only indicates disease of the superficial femoral artery while claudication of the thigh and calf together suggests an occlusion of iliac arteries. Buttock claudication occurs when there is occlusion of the internal iliac artery.
- Claudicants may use different terms to describe the discomfort associated with ambulation and activity like; "cramping", "aching", "weakness", "tightness" and "giving out" (Wright, 1996). This symptom is a result of reduced blood flow and inability of the collateral circulation to meet the oxygen demands of the exercising muscle.
- Approximately 10% of patients will progress to critical ischaemia (see Section 1.1).

- Chronic LLI can be classified into the following stages according to Fontaine's classification:
  - Stage I: Asymptomatic
  - Stage II: Intermittent claudication
  - Stage III: Ischaemic rest pain
  - Stage IV: Ulceration or gangrene, or both.

Signs

- In many patients there may be no significant skin changes. However, in some patients there may be evidence of hair loss or the skin may look dry and scaly.
- The affected limb may feel slightly cooler than the normal limb.
- Pulses in the leg and foot may be reduced or absent. It s important to remember that patients with isolated stenotic lesions may have normal pulses at rest and it is only after exercise that the pulses become reduced or absent (Table 1.1.3).

Assessment

Assessment of patients with PAD should include the following:

- History of the presenting illness.
- Social history.
- History of risk factors: cardiac, diabetes, hypertension and hyper-cholestraemia.
- Physical examination: a part from routine general examination a thorough examination of the legs should be conducted. This should include inspection to detect any trophic changes as well as palpation of all pulses.

Table 1.1.3: Clinical features of LLI

Symptoms
- Pain in calf, thigh, buttock, brought on by exercise and relieved by rest
- Walking distance is limited
- Numbness, pins and needles in skin of the foot
- Impotence in patients with aorto-iliac disease
- Symptoms of coronary or cerebrovascular atherosclerosis, i.e. angina, TIAs

Signs in affected leg
- Affected leg may feel cooler
- Diminished peripheral pulses, or absent distal to level of involved segment

- If the pain is atypical, a full examination of the lumbar spine, hip and knee joints should also be done to exclude spinal stenosis and osteoarthritis as a cause of the patient's symptoms.
- No vascular examination is complete without recording the ankle brachial pressure index (ABPI).

The ankle brachial pressure index

- The ABPI is an inexpensive, non-invasive diagnostic test that is both highly sensitive and specific for PAD, and this test can quantitatively clarify the severity of PAD in nearly all affected individuals, whether symptomatic or not.
- The ABPI is also an accurate predictor of poor prognosis.
- Patients with an ABPI of 0.90 or less are diagnosed to have PVD. It is important to note that an ABPI can be difficult to measure in patients with long-standing diabetes or other older patients with calcified calf arteries, not compressible by the blood pressure cuff.

How to record the ankle brachial pressure index

- Rest the patient in a supine position.
- Measure the systolic blood pressure in both arms.
- Measure the ankle systolic blood pressure from the left and right dorsalis pedis (DP) and posterior tibial (PT) arteries.
- The value of one ankle is taken from the higher of the DP and PT readings.
- The ABPI is calculated by dividing the highest ankle pressure by the highest brachial pressure (McKenna et al., 1991) (Figure 1.1.2).

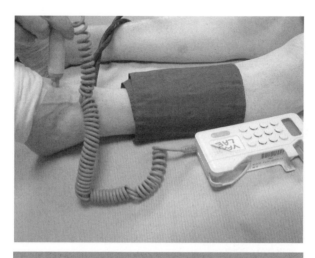

Fig. 1.1.2: Recording the ABPI.

ABPI interpretation

ABPI measurements and interpretations are given in Table 1.1.4.

Table 1.1.4: ABPI interpretation	
Measurement	**Interpretation**
Above 0.90	Normal
0.71–0.90	Mild obstruction
0.41–0.70	Moderate obstruction
0.00–0.40	Severe obstruction

Investigations

- Colour duplex is the first line of investigation. It provides a non-invasive means of localising the disease (please see Chapter 3.1).
- Angiography is usually considered when intervention is contemplated (please see Chapter 3.2).

Management

- Once the assessment is completed, the vascular team summarises the findings and devises a management plan for the patient.
- For patients with intermittent claudication the treatment is essentially conservative. This will include the management of risk factors (see above) and exercise.
- Younger patients with disabling claudications especially if it is affecting lifestyle or jobs may require intervention. (For radiological intervention please refer to Chapter 3.2 and for surgical revascularisation please see Chapter 5.3).

Treatment options for intermittent claudication

Treatment options for intermittent claudication are given in Table 1.1.5.

Prognosis

- The majority of patients (approximately 70%) will improve with conservative treatment.
- Symptoms will deteriorate in <30%.
- About 10% will progress to critical ischaemia.
- Between 2% and 4% patients will require amputation.
- Thirty per cent of claudicants will die within 5 years and 50% within 10 years. The commonest cause of death is ischaemic heart disease (50%), while cerebro-vascular accounts for 15% of death.

Table 1.1.5: Treatment options for intermittent claudication

Treatment 1	• Medical management
	  – Risk factor modification
	  – Exercise programme

Treatment 2	• Radiological management
	  – Risk factor modification
	  – Duplex scan
	  – Peripheral angiography and
	    angioplasty

Treatment 3	• Surgical management
	  – Risk factor modification
	  – Bypass procedure

CRITICAL LIMB ISCHAEMIA

Critical limb ischaemia (CLI) is defined as a state in which the blood supply to the leg is so compromised that its survival is threatened.

The term CLI should only be used in relation to chronic limb ischaemia and should be distinguished from acute limb ischaemia (see Chapter 2).

It indicates a severe and advanced ischaemia that requires urgent action to salvage the affected limb.

Clinical features

- Rest pain which is defined as a persistently recurring pain requiring regular analgesia for more than 2 weeks. It is usually burning in nature and affects the toes and the forefoot. It is worse at night and often eased by hanging the foot out of bed.
- Skin colour ranges from pallor to cyanosis.
- Ulceration on toes or foot and tissue loss.
- Gangrene is defined as dead tissues associated with putrefaction. It may become infected and produces a foul smell.
- Skin blisters may be present.
- Ankle systolic pressure of 50 mmHg or less (in non-diabetics) or a toe systolic pressure of 30 mmHg or less (in diabetics) (Figure 1.1.3).

Management

- The primary aim of the management is to salvage the limb, relieve symptoms and restore function. However, it is important to remember that very

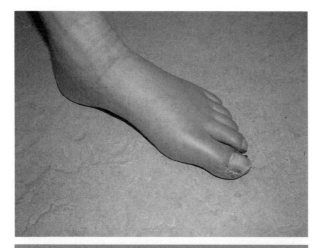

Fig. 1.1.3: Critical ischaemia of left leg. Note the dusky colour and early gangrenous changes of the big toe.

often these are very unfit for patients with many other co-morbidities and the general condition of the patient will dictate the course of treatment.

- Full assessment of the patient is mandatory. This will include history, clinical examination and investigations.
- Associated risk factors like hypertension, hypercholestraemia, smoking and diabetes should be attended to.
- Diabetes is a particularly important risk factor because it is frequently associated with severe arterial disease. Furthermore, atherosclerosis affects the more distal vessels in patients with diabetes which are less amenable to revascularisation. As a result diabetic patients have a higher rate of amputation.
- Infection should be treated with appropriate antibiotics.
- While Duplex scan can identify and localise the sites of the occlusions, angiography is usually performed for further evaluation and planning of intervention.
- Angioplasty has assumed a major role in the treatment of CLI and produced results which are comparable to surgery. It is best suited for stenosis or short lesions of the iliac or superficial femoral artery. Subintimal angioplasty has been shown to produce good results with long occlusions.
- Angioplasty has the added advantage of shorter hospital stay and lower mortality than surgery.
- For many years, surgical revascularisation has been the main treatment option. However, it is limited by the fact that bypasses to the tibial vessels is possible in 30% of cases only. It also carries a significant mortality.

REFERENCES

Antiplatelet Trialists' Collaboration (1988) Secondary prevention of vascular disease by prolonged antiplatelet treatment. *Br Med J* 296: 320–331.

Beach KW, Bedford GR *et al.* (1988) Progression of lower-extremity arterial occlusive disease in type II diabetes mellitus. *Diabetes Care* 11: 464.

Beard JD (2000) Chronic lower limb ischaemia. *Br Med J* 320: 854–857.

Beks PJ *et al.* (1995) Peripheral arterial disease in relation to glycaemic level in an elderly Caucasian population: the Hoorn study. *Diabetologia* 38: 86–96.

Belch JJF, McArdle B, Burns P *et al.* (1984) The effects of acute smoking on platelet behaviour, fibrinolysis and haemorrheology in habitual smokers. *Thromb Res* 51: 6–8.

Bradman O, Redisch W (1953) Incidence of peripheral vascular changes in diabetes mellitus: a survey of 264 cases. *Diabetes* 2(3).

British Hypertension Society Guidelines (1999) *Br Med J* 319: 630–635.

CAPRIE Steering Committee (1996) A randomised, blinded trial of clopidogrel versus aspirin in patients at risk of ischaemic events (CAPRIE). *Lancet* 348: 1329–1339.

Colwell JA (1987) Atherosclerosis in diabetes mellitus. In: Alberti & Krall (eds). *The Diabetes Annual/3*. Elsevier Science Publishers, New York; p. 325.

Fowkes, Dunbar & Lee (1995) Risk factor profile of non-smokers with peripheral arterial disease. *Angiology* 46: 657–662.

Hughson WG, Mann JI & Garrod A (1978) Intermittent claudication: prevalence and risk factors. *Br Med J* 1: 1379.

Kannel WB (1996) The demographics of claudication and the ageing of the American population. *Vasc Med* 1: 60–64.

Kannel WB & McGee DL (1985) Update on some epidemiological features of inter-mittent claudication: the Framingham Study. *J Am Geriat Soc* 22: 13.

Krupski WC (1991) The peripheral vascular consequences of smoking. *Ann Vasc Surg* 5(3): 33–345.

Leng GC, Fowler B & Ernst E (2001) Exercise for intermittent claudication. *The Cochrane Library*, issue 2.

Levy LA (1989) Smoking and peripheral vascular disease. Epidemiology and podiatric perspective. *J Am Pediatr Med Assoc* 79: 398–402.

Lowe GD *et al.* (1991) Blood viscosity, fibrinogen and activation of coagulation and leucocytes in peripheral arterial disease: the Edinburgh Artery Study. *Br J Haematol* 7(Suppl 1): 12–17.

Matsumura JS (1999) Surgery of the aorta. In: Fahey VA (ed.). *Vascular Nursing*, 3rd Edition. WB Saunders Co, Philadelphia; pp. 212–232.

McKenna M, Wolfson S & Kuller L (1991) The ratio of ankle and arm arterial pressure as an independent predictor of mortality. *Atherosclerosis* 87(2–3): 119–128.

Mikhailidis DP (2000) Cardiovascular risk factors in patients with peripheral vascular disease Chapter 1. In: Baker D (ed.). *Primary Care of Vascular Disease*; pp. 1–4.

Schroll M & Munck O (1981) Estimation of peripheral atherosclerosic disease by ankle brachial pressure measurements in a population study of 60-year-old men and women. *J Chronic Dis* 34: 261–269.

Shearman CP (2002) Management of intermittent claudication. *Br J Surg* 89: 529–531.

Shearman CP & Chulakadabba A (1999) The value of risk factor management in patients with peripheral arterial disease. In: *The Evidence for Vascular Surgery*, Chapter 5, tfm Publishing Ltd, Shropshire.

Smith FB *et al.* (1993) Smoking, haemostatic factors and lipid peroxides in a population case control study of peripheral arterial disease. *Atherosclerosis* 102: 155–162.

Strano A *et al.* (1993) Hypertension and other risk factors in peripheral arterial disease. *Clin Exp Hypertens* 15: 71–89.

Wright D (1996) Evaluation of the patient with peripheral vascular disease. In: Demeter S, Andersson G & Smith G (eds). *Disability Evaluation*. St. Louis (MO) Mosby; pp. 367–377.

1.2   CAROTID ARTERY DISEASE

S. Dorgan and H. Al-Khaffaf

The carotid arteries arise from the aortic arch and carry blood to the head and brain. Atherosclerosis may narrow or block these arteries, and this may present as either an asymptomatic bruits (only detected on clinical examination) or a stroke (Figure 1.2.1 and Table 1.2.1).

A stroke (cerebrovascular accident) is a sudden disruption of the blood flow to the brain. This can be either due to embolism or thrombosis (ischaemic

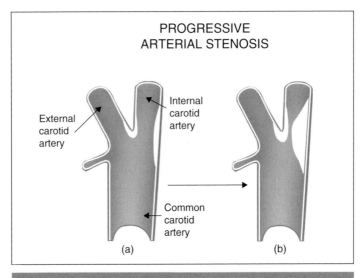

Fig. 1.2.1: Progression of stenosis of the carotid artery.

Table 1.2.1: Carotid artery risk factors	
Modifiable risk factors	**Non-modifiable risk factors**
• Smoking • Cholesterol • Hypertension • Obesity • Lack of exercise	• Age • Gender

stroke) which accounts for about 80% of strokes or bleeding into the brain (haemorrhagic stroke).

The fact that carotid artery disease accounts for approximately over half of all strokes means that surgery can play a major role in stroke prevention.

The symptoms and signs of a stroke depend on the part of the brain affected. There may be a loss or impairment of speech, paralysis of part or all of one side of the body, or loss of balance or muscle coordination. It lasts more than 24 h or leads to death.

If it lasts less than 24 h with a complete recovery it is called a transient ischaemic attack (TIA). A TIA is extremely significant as it is a warning sign of a stroke.

Amaurosis fugax is one form of TIA and refers to blindness or loss of vision in one eye. This sometimes seems like a curtain shade being drawn down over the eye (see Tables 1.2.2 and 1.2.3).

Table 1.2.2: Prognosis: risk of developing a full CVA following a TIA or stroke treated medically

% CVA following	Within 1 year (%)	Yearly after 1 year (%)	Within 5 years (%)
TIA	8.5	5	29
CVA	9	9	45

CVA: cerebrovascular accident.
Ref.: cited by Baker, 2000. In: *Primary Care of Vascular Disease*

Table 1.2.3: Treatment options for carotid artery disease

Treatment 1	• Medical management – Risk factor modification – Anti-platelet medication – Review – outpatients
Treatment 2	• Radiological management – Risk factor modification – Anti-platelet medication – Carotid artery duplex scan – Angioplasty ± stenting
Treatment 3	• Surgical management – Risk factor modification – Anti-platelet medication – Carotid artery duplex ± angiography – Carotid endarterectomy

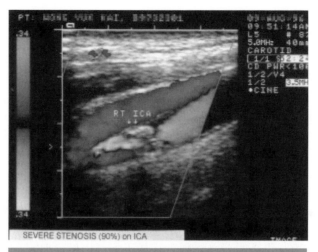

Fig. 1.2.2: Duplex scan of a stenosed internal carotid artery.

Investigations

- *Duplex scan* is the investigation of choice. It can localise the stenosis, identify the degree of the stenosis and characterise the plaque at the carotid bifurcation (see Chapter 3.1) (Figure 1.2.2).
- *Carotid angiography* although it remains the gold standard it is only considered if the Duplex scan result is equivocal (Figure 1.2.4). Please see Chapter 3.2.
- *CT angiography* has proved to be pretty accurate in identifying stenosis and can be used as an adjunct to Duplex scan when it is inconclusive (Figure 1.2.3).
- *MRI scans.*

Indications for carotid endarterectomy

- Patients with symptomatic ipsilateral carotid stenosis >80% benefit from carotid endarterectomy (six operations will prevent one stroke) (Perkins & Galland, 1999).
- There is no advantage from surgery over best medical therapy in patients with symptomatic ipsilateral carotid stenosis <70%.
- Patients with asymptomatic carotid stenosis >75% have reduced risk of stroke after carotid endarterectomy, but the advantage is marginal (50 operations will prevent one stroke).

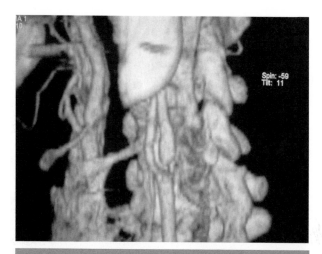

Fig. 1.2.3: Spiral CT angiogram showing a very tight stenosis at the origin of the internal carotid artery.

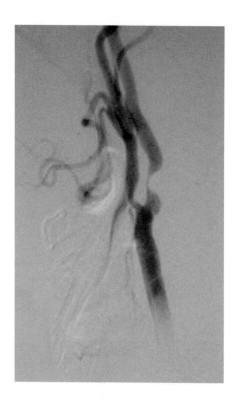

Fig. 1.2.4: Carotid angiogram showing a tight stenosis of the internal carotid artery.

REFERENCE

Perkins & Galland (1999) Indications for carotid endarterectomy: lessons learned from randomised trials. Chapter 1. In: *The Evidence for Vascular Surgery*. TFM Publishing limited, Shropshire.

1.3 ABDOMINAL AORTIC ANEURYSM

S. Dorgan and H. Al-Khaffaf

An abdominal aortic aneurysm (AAA) is a localised permanent dilatation of the aorta. The normal diameter of the abdominal aorta is approximately 2.5 cm (1 inch) (Figure 1.3.1).

When a vessel has a diameter 50% greater than would be expected for a patient's age and sex, it is classified as aneurysmal. However, the abdominal aorta is deemed aneurysmal when its external diameter exceeds 3.0 cm.

AAA affects 5% of men over the age of 65 years and causes 2% of all death in this age group.

It accounts for around 6000 deaths per year in England and Wales.

The natural history of an aneurysm is that it will grow larger and eventually rupture if it is not diagnosed and treated.

Less than half of those with rupture reach hospital and only around 50% of these patients survive emergency surgery.

Aneurysms can:

1. rupture, causing pain, internal haemorrhage and shock;
2. thrombose, leading to acute ischaemia of all downstream branches;
3. embolise, causing selective branch vessel symptoms.

The most common place to find an aneurysm is in the abdominal aorta, but they can also be present in the popliteal artery, thoracic aorta and cerebral area. Twenty-five per cent of patients have aneurysmal disease elsewhere in the iliac, femoral or popliteal arteries. Ninety-five per cent of AAA occurs below the renal arteries.

Aetiology

- The aetiology of AAA is complex and is not fully understood. Current evidence suggests that it is caused by an interplay of environmental and genetic factors (Tilson & Boyd (eds), 1996).
- The four main risk factors are smoking, age (rare before age 55), male sex and family history.

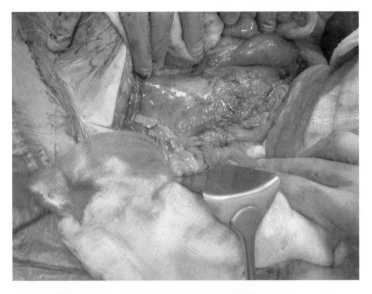

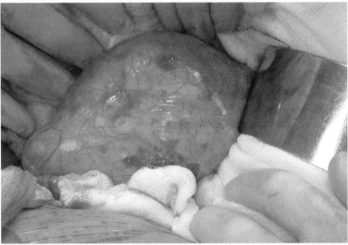

Fig. 1.3.1: Aortic aneurysm.

- Although atherosclerosis is a common feature of AAA its exact role is not well understood, as it is primarily a disease of the intima while aneurysm formation mainly affects the media and adventitia.
- It has been suggested that the enzymes matrix metalloproteinase proteinases (MMPs) play a significant part in aneurysm formation.
- In some patients AAA may be associated with a dense retroperitoneal fibrosis (inflammatory aneurysms), the cause of which is unknown.

Clinical features

Many people can have an aortic aneurysm for many years before developing any symptoms. Symptoms vary according to the location and type of the aneurysm.

Symptoms
- Sixty per cent are asymptomatic.
- Pulsatile feeling in the abdomen.
- Low back or abdominal pain.
- Acute limb ischaemia if thrombus embolises distally.

Signs
- Midline supra-umbilical swelling, i.e. expansile and pulsatile.
- AAA may not be palpable in obese patients or following rupture.
- Rupture usually presents as shock and circulatory collapse in patients with abdominal or back pain.

Diagnosis

AAA are often found on routine physical examination, and chest and abdominal X-rays. It is not uncommon for the patient to be undergoing examination for another medical problem (e.g. urological or orthopaedic) when an AAA is found.

On examination, a pulsating mass in the abdomen may be felt. If an aneurysm is suspected, an ultrasound scan will be performed (Figure 1.3.2). Scans such as computerised tomography (CT) and magnetic resonance imaging (MRI) may also be performed to establish the location of the AAA in relation to the renal and iliac arteries (Figure 1.3.3).

Prognosis

- AAA tend to enlarge and eventually rupture (see Chapter 2).
- It expands at about 10% per year with the rate of expansion increasing as size increases.
- The risk of rupture is mainly related to aneurysm diameter. Other factors associated with rupture include diastolic blood pressure, smoking, chronic obstructive airway disease (COAD) and family history.

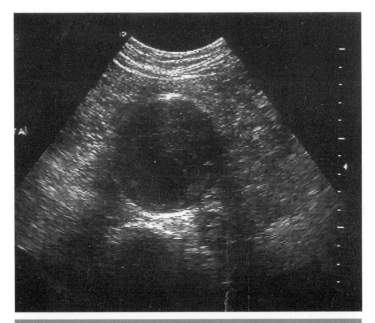

Fig. 1.3.2: Ultrasound scan of AAA showing its tranverse diameters.

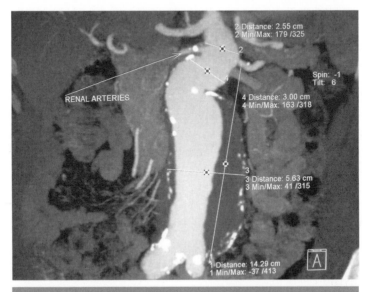

Fig. 1.3.3: CT scan of AAA.

- Five year risk of rupture in relation to diameter:
  - 5.0–5.9 cm is 25%,
  - 6.0–6.9 cm is 35%,
  - >7 cm is 75%.
- It is interesting to note that many patients with AAA die from an unrelated cause rather than the aneurysm itself.

Treatment options

Treatment options for AAA are given in Table 1.3.1.

Endovascular aneurysm repair

- More recently a minimally invasive endovascular alternative to open repair of AAA has been available at certain vascular centres for selected patients. Within this procedure, laparotomy and aortic cross-clamping are avoided as a covered stent-graft is inserted via the femoral arteries (see Chapter 3) (Figure 1.3.4).
- A national randomised multi-centre trial (endovascular aneurysm repair, EVAR) is underway to compare endovascular repair and open surgical repair, and is due to report its results soon.

Aneurysm screening

Screening of aortic aneurysm has appealed to many vascular surgeons because:

- Many aneurysms remain asymptomatic until they suddenly rupture with a high mortality rate.
- A simple non-invasive ultrasound scan can detect 99% of asymptomatic AAA.

Table 1.3.1: Treatment options for AAA	

Treatment 1	• Medical management
	  – Risk factor modification
	  – Duplex scan and aneurysm surveillance

Treatment 2	• Elective repair if
	  – AAA >5.5 cm
	  – Rapidly expanding AAA (>1.0 cm in 6/12)
	  – Tender AAA

Treatment 3	• Emergency repair if
	  – Collapse
	  – Abdominal/back pain
	  – Pulsatile abdominal mass (which signifies ruptured AAA)

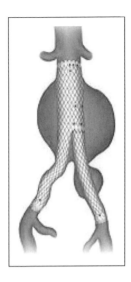

Fig. 1.3.4: Diagram of an aortic stent.

- Elective treatment is very effective with good long-term results and a low mortality rate.

While this may appear to be logical, the argument against screening has been focused on the cost-effectiveness of a national aneurysm-screening programme. However, the recently published results of the MASS trial (multicentre aneurysm-screening study) have shown that a single ultrasound scan at the age of 65 years with a subsequent repair of AAA over 5.5 cm in diameter reduces the risk of death from a ruptured AAA by 42%. It has also confirmed that it is cost-effective. The annual cost of a national screening programme for the UK would be less than £15 millions, falling to less than £5 millions within 10 years.

REFERENCES

Beard JD (2003) Screening for abdominal aortic aneurysm (Leading article). *Br J Surg* 90: 515–516.

Brown LC & Powell JT, for the UK small aneurysm trial participants (1999) Risk factors for aneurysm rupture in patients kept under ultrasound surveillance. UK small aneurysm trial participants. *Ann Surg* 230: 289–297.

Greenhalgh R & Powell J (2002) Screening men for aortic aneurysm. *Br Med J* 325: 1123.

Multicentre Aneurysm Screening Study Group (2002) Multicentre aneurysm screening study (MASS): cost effectiveness analysis of screening for abdominal aortic aneurysms based on four year results from a randomised controlled trial. *Br Med J* 325: 1135–1138.

Tilson MD & Boyd CD (eds) (1996) The abdominal aortic aneurysm: genetics, pathophysiology, molecular biology. *Ann NY Acad Sci* 800: New York, NY.

1.4 UPPER LIMB ISCHAEMIA

H. Al-Khaffaf

In comparison to the lower limb, ischaemia of the upper limb is uncommon and accounts for <5% of patients with limb ischaemia.

Aetiology: Acute upper limb ischaemia accounts for approximately 15% of all acute lower and upper limb ischaemia. Causes include embolism, trauma and iatrogenic injuries like cardiac catheterisation and intra-arterial drug abuse. (see Chapter 2).

Chronic ischaemia due to atherosclerosis is rare mainly due to the good collateral circulation around the shoulder that compensate for the stenosis or occlusion and therefore many patients remain asymptomatic (Figure 1.4.1).

Although atherosclerosis can affect any part of the arterial tree, certain sections like the proximal subclavian artery are more commonly affected producing what is clinically known as the subclavian steal syndrome (SSS).

Patients with SSS may have episodes of dizziness or ipsilateral arm claudiacation.

Clinical examination will show a weak or absent ipsilateral radial pulse with a reduced blood pressure compared to the contra-lateral arm.

Diagnosis can be confirmed with a Duplex scan but angiography may be required in certain cases where Duplex is inconclusive (Figure 1.4.2).

Balloon angioplasty is the treatment of choice and is only indicated when symptoms are disabling or interfering with the patient's lifestyle.

Acute	Chronic
• Embolism	• Atherosclerosis
• Trauma	• Raynaud's disease
• Iatrogenic	• Arteritis
	• Thoracic outlet syndrome
	• Thrombophilia

Fig. 1.4.1: Causes of upper limb ischaemia.

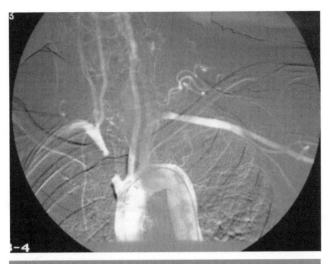

Fig. 1.4.2: An aortic arch angiogram showing a complete occlusion of the innominate artery.

Bypass surgery is rarely needed but can be considered when angioplasty is unsuccessful. Carotid-subclavian bypass is the most commonly used technique.

REFERENCES

Bhasker S & Scott DJA (1999–2000) Upper limb Ischaemia, vascular surgery highlights. Daryl Baker Primary care of vascular disease.
http://www.emedicine.com/radio/topic663.htm

1.5. RAYNAUD'S PHENOMENON

S. Dorgan

Raynaud's phenomenon (RP) is a common, episodic circulatory disorder and the term is used to describe the spasm of the arteries supplying the acral parts of the body (in particular the fingers and toes).

It is often precipitated by cold and relieved by heat (Macleod, 1974) and is different from chilblains or permanently cold, blue or white hands.

Trauma, hormones and chemicals can also provoke an attack (Belch, 1990).

RP may be severe for some sufferers and indicative of an underlying disorder, however, few patients who have this disorder seek help for their symptoms.

Pathophysiology

Understanding the normal anatomy of the arteries and the physiology of vasoconstriction helps explain how this phenomenon occurs:

- Arteries are made up of three common layers and the structure of them enable elasticity and contractility, and any alterations in blood pressure is permitted by passive changes in vessel diameter.
- Contractility allows arteries to change in diameter under nervous and humoral control (this is control via substances absorbed or secreted into the body fluid, such as hormones).
- Vasoconstriction results from stimulation and relaxation results in vaso-dilation (Guyton & Hall, 1996; Martini, 1998). Arterioles are the end branches of the arterial tree and supply the capillary bed, and it is the arterioles that are primarily affected in RP.
- It appears that in RP there is an abnormal response of the peripheral arterioles to normal constrictive and dilatational mechanisms, which causes prolonged digital artery vasospasm (Roath, 1986).

Clinical manifestations

RP is manifest by pallor of the digits, followed by cyanosis and rubor:

- The pallor reflects vasospasm in the digital vessels (white).

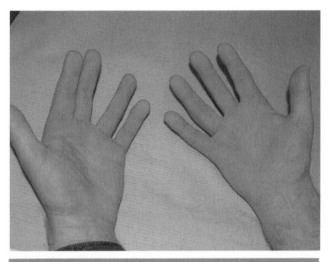

Fig. 1.5.1: Reactive hyperaemia in a patient with Raynaud's disease.

- Deoxygenation of static venous return results in cyanosis (blue).
- Reactive hyperaemia following return of blood flow causes rubor (red) (Figure 1.5.1).
- It should be noted that the full triphasic colour change is not essential for diagnosis (Belch, 1990) although cyanosis, pallor or both should occur episodically.
- In addition, tingling and numbness of the fingers are usual concurrent symptoms.
- Attacks can vary in their duration, some lasting for hours (Kumar & Clark, 1998) and sufferers may notice that spasms become gradually more frequent and prolonged.
- Recovery often begins at the base of the fingers when the pale digits return to a bright red colour and pain can be severe with a burning sensation in the fingers in the re-warming phase. Intense rubor, parathesia, throbbing and swelling may also occur (Krupp & Chatton, 1975).
- Attacks of RP usually end as a result of the person:
  – immersing the affected part in warm water,
  – returning to a warm room,
  – spontaneously.

It is essential to note that a diagnosis of RP is not automatically given to a person experiencing white numb fingers, having chilblains or feeling constantly cold.

Primary and secondary Raynaud's phenomenon

RP can be differentiated into primary and secondary:

- Primary RP can occur without any underlying disease and be no more than an exaggerated physiological response to cold. In this case it is usually benign.
- Secondary RP, which is less common, is where there is an associated disorder (such as scleroderma and systemic lupus erythematosus). Somewhat confusing is that this classification applies only in Europe and health care professionals in the USA may use the words "syndrome" and "phenomenon" interchangeably. Differentiating between primary and secondary RP is essential as treating any underlying disease may improve the symptoms of RP.

Investigations

- Full blood count with erythrocyte sedimentation rate (ESR).
- Urea and electrolytes/liver function tests.
- Creatinine phosphokinase.
- C-reactive protein (CRP).
- Antinuclear antibodies.
- Chest X-ray with thoracic inlet view if patient has unilateral Raynaud's.

Treatment

There are ways of improving the condition even though it cannot be cured and treatment will depend on the underlying condition and the severity of the attack. Primary RP is most probably multifactorial, which means it is not necessary for all patients with RP to undergo the same pathophysiological changes. This would suggest that suitability of treatments vary between patients, though drug therapy can often be avoided for those people with mild forms of the disease. Recommendations at this stage include:

- Stopping smoking (due to its effect on the microcirculation).
- Cessation of taking drugs with a known association with RP.
- Change in occupation.
- Keeping the body warm. Heat treatment can help reduce pain and muscle stiffness.
- Protection of hands from exposure to the cold.
- Wearing gloves in the cold. However, gloves may be uncomfortable to wear and carry around.
- Stopping taking the contraceptive pill if there is a definite link with the development of the disease (Belch, 1990).

Drug therapy

There is some controversy regarding the benefit of vasodilators to treat RP as much of the research constitutes uncontrolled studies. Drug schemes that are used in the treatment of RP include nifedipine, stanozolol (stromba), inositol nicotinate (hexopal), naftidrofuryl oxalate (praxilene) and prostaglandin 12. Vasodilators (such as calcium channel blocker) aim to increase the blood flow in the affected areas, but their value is limited. Side effects (headaches) may result if relatively large doses of medication are required (Sturgill & Seibold, 1998). Despite the varied opinions regarding vasodilators for this condition, it is agreed that regular analgesia is essential when the person experiences pain.

Surgical intervention

Local sympathectomy may play a role when attacks are frequent or significantly impact on working life. This procedure attempts to cut off the sympathetic outflow to the hands and aims to improve the blood flow to the hands up to a certain point. Unfortunately, high relapse rates are often associated with this treatment option (Lau & Belch, 1991).

Role of the nurse

The aim of the nurse is to enable the person and their family to accept their condition, and adopt a positive coping strategy.

- Patients need advice on how to maintain a constant body temperature.
- Reassurance is essential as this disease can evoke apprehension in its sufferers.
- A self-help group,"The Raynaud's Association" offers education, support and advice, and patients should be informed of its existence.
- Advice on how to protect themselves from the cold should also be given to patients: purchasing electrically-heated socks and gloves, shoes designed to keep feet warm and relieve pressure on the toes may offer some comfort.
- Advice on stress and anxiety reducing activities is essential as in primary Raynaud's, up to a third of vasospastic attacks have been triggered by stress (Freedman & Ianni, 1983). Thus, the nurse may recommend exercise such as walking and swimming to aid feelings of calm.
- Education regarding other triggers which include touching cold objects, slight change in temperature or going into a cold atmosphere.
- The patient should be encouraged to be active in self-care management.
- Each person needs to be considered individually, and assessed physically, socially and psychologically (Figure 1.5.2).

• Arthritis	• Skin rashes
• Alopecia	• Weight loss
• Respiratory/cardiac problems	• Dry eyes/mouth
• Absent pulses	• Photosensitivity
• Muscle weakness	• Oral ulceration
• Cerebral symptoms	• Blood pressure
• Finger ulcers	• Oesophageal symptoms
• Changes in skin texture	

Fig. 1.5.2: A table of the signs and symptoms of underlying disease in patients presenting with Raynaud's.

For further information on Raynaud's phenomenon contact:

Raynaud's & Scleroderma Association, 112 Crewe Road, Alsagar, Cheshire, ST7 2JA (Tel: 01270 872776/Fax: 01270 883556).

REFERENCES

Belch JJF (1990) Management of Raynaud's phenomenon, Hospital Update May: 391–400.

Freedman RR & Ianni P (1983) Role of cold and emotional stress in Raynaud's disease & scleroderma. *Br Med J* 287: 1499–1502.

Guyton AC & Hall JE (1996) In: *Textbook of Medical Physiology*, 9th Edition. WB Saunders, London.

Krupp MA & Chatton MJ (1975) *Current Medical Diagnosis & Treatment*. Lange Medical Publications, Los Altos, California.

Kumar P & Clark M (1998) *Clinical Medicine*, 4th Edition. WB Saunders, London.

Lau CS & Belch JJF (1991) Raynaud's phenomenon – a vasospastic disorder. *Curr Pract Surg* 3: 170–175.

Macleod J (1974) *Davidson's Principles & Practice of Medicine*, 11th Edition. Churchill Livingstone, London.

Martini FH (1998) *Fundamentals of Anatomy & Physiology*, 4th Edition. Prentice Hall, New Jersey.

Roath OS (1986) Managing Raynaud's phenomenon. *Br Med J* 293: 88–89.

Sturgill MG & Seibold JR (1998) Rational use of calcium channel antagonists in Raynaud's phenomenon. *Curr Opin Rheumatol* 10: 584–588.

1.6   VASCULITIS

S. Dorgan and H. Al-Khaffaf

Definition

Vasculitis is a general term for a group of diseases that involve inflammation of the blood vessels. Any type and size of vessel may be involved: Arteries, arterioles, veins, venules and capillaries. However, it is generally classified into:

- large-vessel vasculitis,
- medium-vessel vasculitis,
- small-vessel vasculitis.

Causes of vasculitis

The causes of vasculitis are unknown. While infection with bacteria, viruses or fungi can cause vasculitis, the majority of cases are the result of an immune reaction. As a result of an unknown stimulus the immune system becomes hyperactive and leads to inflammations in different body tissues including blood vessels. This in turn will lead to narrowing of the affected blood vessels.

Symptoms

Vasculitis may be localised or systemic. Many organs and different parts of the body may be affected. Thus, many different symptoms may occur as a result of vasculitis, depending on the severity of the tissue damage and what tissues are involved. The lack of blood supply may cause necrosis, thrombosis or an aneurysm. There are approximately 20 different disorders that are classified as "vasculitis". Two of the these disorders that may be seen in vascular practice are briefly described below.

BUERGER'S DISEASE (THROMBOANGIITIS OBLITERANS)

- Buerger's disease is an inflammatory disease of the small- and medium-sized arteries and veins of the extremities.
- First described by Buerger in 1908.
- Patients are usually heavy smokers young males aged 20–40 years.
- Most common in Southeast Asia, India and the Middle East.

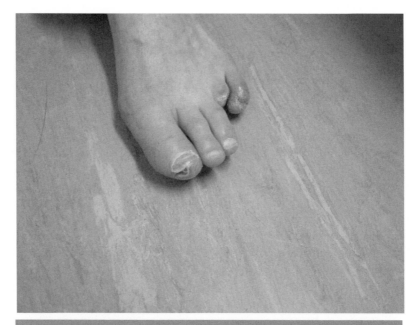

Fig. 1.6.1: Early gangrenous changes of toes in a patient with Buerger's disease. Note the already amputated 4th toe.

- Symptoms include intermittent claudication, numbness, rest pain, ulcers and gangrene of the digits (fingers and toes) (see Figure 1.6.1).
- Examination usually shows normal proximal pulses and diminished or absent distal pulses.
- Diagnosis is confirmed by angiography. It is important to exclude other conditions that may mimic Buerger's disease such as atherosclerosis and severe Raynaud's disease.
- Treatment: The only known effective treatment is cessation of smoking. Anti-inflammatory agents such as steroids are of no benefits. Similarly anticoagulants are of little value. Ilioprost infusion may offer some help.
- Patients who continue to smoke may end up having amputation of digits or fingers.

TAKAYASU'S ARTERITIS

- A rare chronic inflammatory condition that affects the aorta and its major branches.
- In contrast to Buerger's disease the typical Takayasu's patient is usually a young female under the age of 40.
- It is more common in Asian women.

- Clinically the disease has two phases: a systemic phase and an occlusive phase.
  - In the systemic phase patients will have constitutional symptoms, i.e. fever, fatigue and weight loss in addition to arthritis and non-specific aches and pains. High erythrocyte sedimentation rate (ESR) is also present in most patients.
  - In the occlusive phase the symptoms are the result of stenosis of the affected arteries. These include claudication of the upper or lower limbs or both. There may be also visual symptoms, headache and dizziness.
- On examination, pulses in the arms or legs may be absent. Blood pressure is often high and there may be bruits over stenosed vessels.
- Diagnosis is often difficult due to the non-specific symptoms that are associated with the early stage of the disease. However, the diagnosis can be confirmed by angiography or MRI scan.
- Treatment: The majority of patients respond well to a course of steroids. For long-term treatment cytotoxic drugs are required.
- Surgery or angioplasty may be required to deal with stenotic lesions.

REFERENCE

http://vasculitis.med.jhu.edu/typesof/buergers.html

S. Dorgan

Definition

The thoracic outlet is the space between the thorax and the clavicle through which the main blood vessels and nerves pass from the neck and thorax into the arm.

Thoracic outlet syndrome (TOS) is a combination of numbness, pain, weakness, tingling or coldness in the upper extremity, which results from pressure on the nerves and/or blood vessels in the thoracic outlet.

Aetiology

- The passageway between the clavicle and first rib has many blood vessels, muscles and nerves.
- If the shoulder muscles in the chest are not able to hold the collarbone in place, it can slip down and forward, which then puts pressure on the nerves and blood vessels that lie under it.
- Symptoms depend on which nerves or blood vessels are being compressed:
  - Pressure on the blood vessels reduces the blood flow to the arm and hands, making them tire easily and feel cool.
  - Pressure on the nerves can result in a vague, aching pain in the neck, shoulder, arm or hand. Overhead activities are especially difficult to perform.

Causes

There are several causes of TOS. It can be as a result of:

- injury,
- disease,
- congenital abnormality,
- poor posture aggravates the condition.

Neurological symptoms

These are more common than the vascular symptoms and include:

- pain,
- numbness,

- tingling,
- arm weakness and poor grip,
- fatigue.

Vascular symptoms

Vascular symptoms include:

- swelling or puffiness in the arm or hand;
- bluish discolouration of the hand;
- coldness in the arm and hand;
- feeling of heaviness in the arm or hand;
- rarely, distal emboli from a subclavian aneurysm.

This syndrome can be difficult to diagnose as the symptoms can mimic many other conditions (such as carpal tunnel syndrome, cervical spondylosis and a herniated disk in the neck).

Diagnosis

Diagnosis can be made from the history and examination. The following investigations can help in establishing the diagnosis:

- Chest X-rays may reveal the presence of a cervical rib.
- Magnetic resonance imaging (MRI) scan can identify a fibrous band compressing nerves and vessels.
- Arch angiography if a subclavian aneurysm is suspected.
- Venography is indicated in cases of subclavian vein thrombosis.

Treatment

This is often conservative. Surgery is not often required. Treatments include:

- Physiotherapy to strengthen the muscles surrounding the shoulder, so that they can support the clavicle.
- A home exercise programme is essential. This should be performed regularly to ensure benefits.
- The length of time the arms are used in outstretched or overhead positions should be reduced.
- Taking frequent breaks, changing positions and stretching are useful.
- Postural exercises to assist patients to sit and stand straighter. This will then lessen the pressure on blood vessels and nerves.

- Non-steroidal and anti-inflammatory drugs to ease the pain.
- Dietary advice if the patient is overweight.
- Strenuous activities should be avoided.
- If conservative treatment is not effective, then surgical intervention may be required. This is often as a last resort, and will involve dividing a muscle in the neck and removing a portion of the first rib.

REFERENCE

http://www.emedicine.com/emerg/topic578.htm

1.8 HYPERHYDROSIS

S. Dorgan and H. Al-Khaffaf

Definition

Hyperhydrosis is excessive sweating. Sweating is a normal bodily process and one of the ways in which the body cools itself. When sweating is excessive and leads to clothes being ruined or social embarrassment it is referred to as *hyperhydrosis*. It is thought that this condition occurs as a result of over activity of the sympathetic nervous system.

Most commonly, hyperhydrosis occurs on the palms of the hands, but it can also occur in the armpits, feet, face and trunk.

Classification

Hyperhydrosis can be either primary or secondary.

Primary hyperhydrosis
- There is no known cause. In some patients there may be a clear family history.
- More common than secondary hyperhydrosis.
- Often localised in one or several areas of the body.
- Affects up to 4% of people.
- Usually starts in childhood or adolescence and persists all life.
- Nervousness and anxiety can aggravate sweating.

Secondary hyperhydrosis
- Hyperhydrosis can occur as a result of certain conditions that can promote excessive sweating.
- Causes include hyperthyroidism, endocrine treatment of prostatic cancer or other types of malignant diseases, severe psychiatric disorders, obesity and menopause.
- Often it involves the whole body.

Manifestations of primary hyperhydrosis

- *Facial hyperhydrosis*: Sweat pouring down from the forehead when stressed can be distressful, leading the patient to feel that other people consider him/her insecure and nervous.
- *Palmar hyperhydrosis*: Excessive sweating of the hands can severely limit individuals in their choice of profession. In extreme cases patients may try

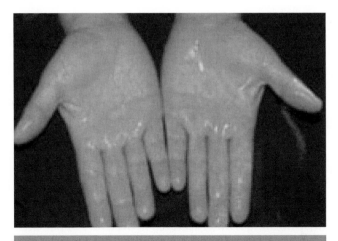

Fig. 1.8.1: Palmar hyperhydrosis.

to avoid social contact. The degree of sweating may range from moderate moisture to dripping (see Figure 1.8.1).

- *Axillary hyperhydrosis*: Sweating of the armpits can cause large wet marks and white salt rings from sweating on clothes.

Management

- Reassurance and psychological support for mild symptoms.
- Prescription of aluminium chloride: a strong antiperspirant, which is applied at night and washed off in the morning.
- Oral anticholinergic agents may be useful in controlling hyperhydrosis but their side effects such as dryness of the mouth and blurring of vision can outweigh their benefits.
- Iontophoresis: which involves the immersion of the hands or feet in a solution and the use of a low intensity electrical current that temporarily disrupts the function of the sweat glands. This will stop sweating for about 4–6 weeks and therefore the process has to be repeated regularly.
- Injection of Botox, a purified protein toxin, can be effective in axillary hyperhydrosis but requires repeated injections every 6–8 months.

If the above measures fail to help, then thoracoscopic sympathectomy may be considered.

Thoracoscopic sympathectomy

- To reduce the amount of sweating, the nerves that supply the sweat glands in the armpit and palms can be cut.

- Using keyhole surgery, the sympathetic chain which lies deep in the upper chest, close to the spine can be destroyed through two or three small holes in the chest.
- When performed by a surgeon experienced in this field, it can produce a definitive cure in nearly all patients.
- A minimal scar may be left in the armpit. (For operative technique please see Chapter 5.3.)

Benefits and risks of a thoracoscopic sympathectomy

Benefits

- Reduction of sweating is often achieved in over 90% of patients. The results are permanent in nearly all cases.
- It is usually more successful for sweating of the palms than the armpits.

Complications

- Pneumothorax: A residue of air can remain between the lung and the chest wall due to either incomplete inflation of the lung or a small leakage from the lung.
- Horner's syndrome: Drooping of the upper eyelid on the side of the operation and pupillary constriction due to damage of sympathetic chain at the level of the stellate ganglion.
- Chest pain at the site of insertion of the telescope. It may last for a few weeks but gradually improves.
- Excessive dryness of the hands can be a problem and may require moisturising of the skin.
- Compensatory hyperhydrosis, mostly over the abdomen and back can be troublesome to many patients. This byfar is the most common complication of sympathectomy, however, the majority of patients can live with it and feel that it is still better than their original problem.

REFERENCE

http://www.emedicine.com/plastic/topic530.htm

1.9 LEG ULCERS

K. Payton and M. Gore

Introduction

The management of leg ulcers represents a significant expense to health services in the UK. Bosanquet (1992) calculated that the cost to the National Health Services (NHS) is estimated in the region of £400 million per annum. Leg ulceration affects 1–2% of the population in the UK, mostly older people (Laing, 1992). Although it is well documented that the majority of care is managed in the community with established leg ulcer clinics and competently trained nurses, a significant number are managed in hospital (University of York, 1997).

Types of leg ulcers

Leg ulcers develop where there is an alteration to the normal physiology. It is important to take time when classifying the ulcer type, due to the many causes of leg ulcer development, as listed below:

- venous disease (approximately 70% of leg ulcers are caused by venous disease);
- arterial disease accounts for approximately 10% of ulceration;
- rheumatoid arthritis;
- diabetes;
- burns;
- lymphoedema;
- malignant disease.

Patient assessment

A full holistic assessment is the most important part of effective leg ulcer management (The Effective Healthcare Bulletin, 1997). Patient assessment is required to determine:

- the immediate cause of the ulcer,
- any underlying pathology in the lower limb,
- other medical problems which may delay healing,
- the patient's social circumstances.

A holistic assessment includes assessment of the following:

- the patient,
- the limb,

- the ulcer,
- the risk factors.

Venous risk factors	Arterial risk factors
• Hypertension	• Smoking
• Phlebitis	• High fat/cholesterol
• Fractures/surgery	• Diet
• Trauma	• Obesity
• Varicose veins	• Sedentary lifestyle
• Multiple pregnancies	• Diabetes
• Immobility	• Rheumatoid arthritis

Venous leg ulcers

These are caused by chronic venous hypertension. The superficial veins are not able to withstand high pressure, the valves become damaged and prevent blood flowing in one direction. The pressure continues to increase in the venules and capillaries. It is in the capillaries that the tissues cannot discharge waste products and deoxygenated blood adequately. This results in a build up of waste products, which causes tissue breakdown. Fibrinogen (protein) passes through the stretched wall into the tissues. The fibrin then combines to form a barrier preventing oxygen and nutrients passing through. The starvation results in tissue death and thus ulcer formation (Figure 1.9.1).

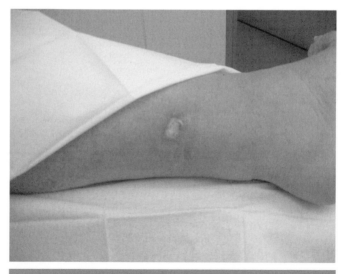

Fig. 1.9.1: A venous ulcer.

Signs and symptoms

Signs and symptoms of venous leg ulcers [adapted from Morison & Moffat, 1994]:

- *Staining of the gaiter area*: This is a brown discolouration which does not resolve. It is caused by red blood cells seeping into the tissues.
- *Ankle flare*: The tiny veins on the medial aspect of the foot become distended.
- *Atrophy of the skin*: A poor blood supply causes thinning of the epidermis.
- *Oedema*: Increased pressure in the capillaries causes them to be tortuous and dilated, fluid leaks into the tissue causing oedema.
- *Eczema*: The non-movement of venous circulation becomes an irritant in the dermal cells producing varicose eczema.
- *Lipodermatosclerosis*: The fibrin deposited at the capillary wall causes the leg to feel hard and woody.
- *Atrophy blanche*: Local areas of capillary infarction can cause loss of pigmentation.

The aim of treating venous ulcers is to:

- reduce blood pressure in the superficial venous system,
- aid the return of venous blood to the heart,
- reduce oedema by reducing the difference in pressure in the capillaries and tissues,
- best way of achieving these aims is to apply **graduated compression bandages**.

Compression therapy

Compression therapy is a means of applying pressure to the limb to promote venous return and lymphatic drainage. Venous leg ulcers can be treated with three or four layer graduated compression bandages or short stretch bandages. Graduated compression is required to aid venous return with 30–40 mmHg at the ankle reducing to 50% of this below the knee. This can be achieved following the shape of the leg (narrower at the ankle than knee). If the ankle is narrow in comparison to the calf (inverted champagne bottle look) extra padding will be required to achieve a "cone" shape (Figures 1.9.2–1.9.8).

Elastic bandages

Elastic bandages apply continuous pressure irrespective of the patients' mobility and position. The elasticity allows them to "give" when the muscle beneath contracts and then return to the original extension. They are applied at 50% extension and usually form part of a three or four layer system (Morrison & Moffat, 1994).

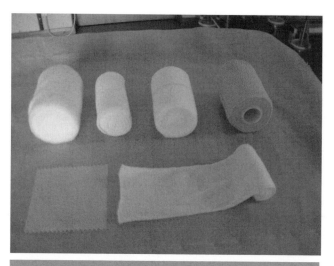

Fig. 1.9.2: Components of four layer compression system.

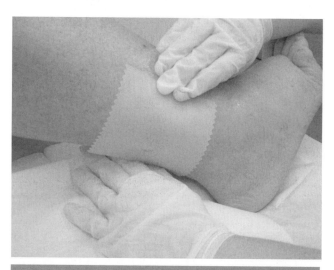

Fig. 1.9.3: 10 cm × 10 cm knitted viscose dressing to protect the wound.

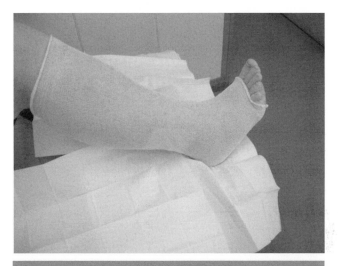

Fig. 1.9.4: A protective stockinette of unbleached cotton is often used to prevent reaction to wool.

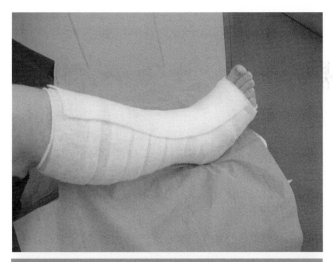

Fig. 1.9.5: Layer 1 of a pure wool or synthetic fibre sub-bandage wadding(10 cm × 2.5 m).This absorbs exudates and redistributes pressure to help prevent damage to bony prominences. Applied in a spiral.

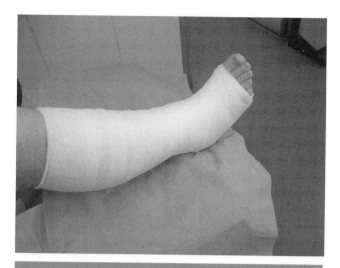

Fig. 1.9.6: Layer 2, consists of a light support bandage (Type2) 10 cm × 4.4 mm. This aids absorbency, maintains the position of the wadding and acts as a base for compression. Applied in a spiral.

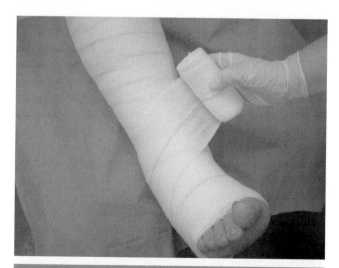

Fig. 1.9.7: Layer 3, a light compression bandage (Type 3a) 10 cm × 6 mm and 10 cm × 8.7 mm. This is the first compression layer and provides 17 mmHg at the ankle. Applied in a figure of eight at 50% stretch.

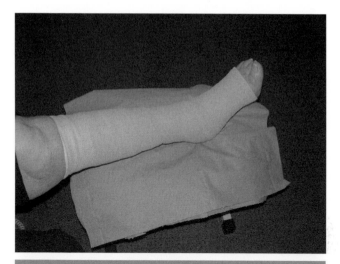

Fig. 1.9.8: Layer 4, a cohesive bandage (Type3a) 10 cm × 6 m. It offers additional compression and provides 23 mmHg at the ankle. Applied in a spiral at 50% stretch.

Inelastic bandages (short stretch)

This bandage is applied at 100% extension and forms an inelastic cuff around the calf which does not yield when the calf muscle contracts. These are most effective when the patient is mobile and useful for patients who may need to carry on with a normal working life as they comprise a two-layer system which is less bulky (Figure 1.9.9).

Accurate measurements of the leg must be taken regularly to ensure the correct bandage regime is used to aid venous return and also to prevent tissue damage from tight bandages. New bandages are brought onto the market continuously so it is important to study the clinical and cost-effectiveness before use. Bandages can be left in place for up to 1 week which ensures continuous pressure over a period of time.

Compression hosiery and aftercare

As leg ulceration is a chronic problem it is important to maintain contact with the patient after the ulcer has healed. Compression hosiery should be worn long term so 3 monthly re-assessments are required to check the status of the circulatory system. Arteries can become compromised in a short time especially in elderly people and it is for this reason that Doppler re-assessment must be carried out regularly.

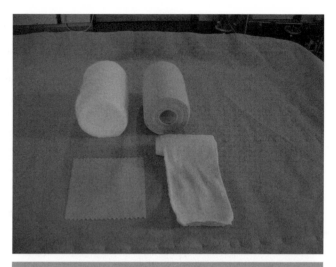

Fig. 1.9.9: Components of short stretch compression system.

The practitioner needs to check that no further ulcers are imminent and that the correct hosiery is being worn. Stockings should be replaced every 3 months as they start to loose their elasticity after this time and become ineffective. Legs also need to be re-measured, as this can change due to weight gain or loss. In some cases compression hosiery can be applied to help heal the ulcer if the patient feels unable to wear bandages. Class III should be worn to aid healing and class II to prevent recurrence.

Advice and education should be offered to the patient on initial assessment and be ongoing throughout the treatment and on re-assessment with regards to caring for the legs long term in order to help prevent recurrence.

Patients should also be advised to wear compression hosiery on the unaffected leg whilst an ulcer is healing to aid even venous return. This has the added affect that the patient becomes familiar with the hosiery and will assist compliance in the future.

It is essential that the patient is given a contact number to discuss any problems that may occur before the next visit is due.

Factors affecting compression
Where pressure exerted by the bandage equates to the:

- number of layers applied,
- tension of the bandage,

- circumference of the limb,
- width of the bandage.

Practitioners must receive training as to the suitability of a particular bandage system and in the correct application. This can only be achieved by practicing application several times under supervision and in some cases using a sub-bandage pressure where available until the correct technique is achieved. It is important that the practitioner has regular update sessions if not carrying out bandaging on a regular basis.

Damage can be caused to limbs by applying bandages inappropriately or too tight or too loose.

Limbs must be measured and observed to ensure that correct bandaging is applied.

Paste bandages can be applied to patients with problematic skin conditions if necessary underneath compression bandages.

Arterial ulcers

These are directly due to insufficient arterial blood supply to the lower limb. This can be caused by either arterial stenosis or blockage:

- Stenosis is caused by atherosclerosis: fatty plaques narrowing the lumen of the artery. Total occlusion can result.
- Blockage is caused by thrombosis which can be attributed to plaque formation also, which can cause fissures and haemorrhages that form into blood clots. This may result in emboli breaking off and lodging in smaller arteries causing sudden breakdown.

Another problem affecting the arteries is arteriosclerosis, when artery walls loose their elasticity and become fibrous, hard and inflexible. The blood flow becomes turbulent, increasing the risk of emboli formation (Figure 1.9.10).

Signs and symptoms
- *Intermittent claudication*: Cramp like pain in the muscle of the leg brought on by walking a certain distance. The patient will stand still for several minutes until the pain is relieved.
- *Rest pain*: Usually when leg is elevated, there is a constant burning pain in the foot, toes and heels. Usually relieved by making the leg dependent, i.e. hanging out of bed or down from an upright chair.
- *Coldness of feet*: Occurring in a patient who does not normally have cold feet.
- *Loss of hair, and atrophic, shiny skin*: On legs due to poor blood supply.

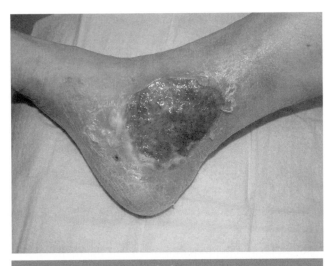

Fig. 1.9.10: An arterial ulcer.

- *Poor tissue profusion*: Colour takes more than 3 s to return after blanching of toe nail bed by applying direct pressure.
- *Colour changes in the feet*: Foot/toes dusky pink turn when dependent, turning pale when raised above the heart.
- *Loss of pedal pulses*: Occasionally pedal pulses cannot be palpated even if there is no arterial problem. Until Doppler assessment or duplex scan is performed a correct diagnosis cannot be obtained.
- *Ulcer appearance*: Small, deep and well-defined ulcers are more likely to have arterial origins.

Treatment

The nurse should try to determine the degree of arterial disease by carrying out a full holistic assessment. This involves simple clinical investigations, along with estimating the ankle brachial pressure index (ABPI) through Doppler assessment. This will provide information for correct referral if appropriate.

Compression bandaging in contraindicated for patients with significant arterial disease.

The aim of treating arterial ulcers
- Keep free from infection.
- Alleviate pain.
- Provide conservative management concerned with the maintenance of the limb with appropriate dressings.

- Prevent deteriorations of the limb by observation, referral if necessary, and health education.
- Provide psychological support.

Wound maintanence

- Topical applications of creams, sprays or antibiotics should not be used as they have no proven value in ulcer healing (Morgan, 1987; Browse *et al.*, 1986).
- Oral antibiotics should be prescribed if clinical infection has been correctly identified.
- Dressings should be applied according to the condition of the wound, bearing in mind the need to control exudates, pain levels and to prevent damage to the surrounding skin.
- Dressings that are non-adherent help to keep pain levels at a minimum on dressing changes.
- Whenever possible, dressings and bandages should be changed before "strike through" of exudates has occurred. This will reduce the risk of bacterial contamination.
- Pain levels should be monitored and effective analgesia prescribed.
- Mild exercise and ankle movements should be encouraged, particularly if the patient is immobile.
- Patients suffering from diabetes mellitus and rheumatoid arthritis commonly develop arterial problems involving small and large blood vessels. Treatment should be closely monitored by nursing and medical staff.

Mixed aetiology ulcers

This group of patients will exhibit both signs and symptoms of arterial and venous disease, and are a difficult category to assess and treat. A thorough holistic assessment must take place. Doppler ultrasound followed by duplex scan may be necessary to estimate the severity of the condition. Three monthly re-assessment should take place as status can change quickly (Simon *et al.*, 1994).

Treatment

Treatment will depend on whether the ulcer is predominantly venous or arterial. The main aims are to:

- Determine the degree of arterial insufficiency.
- Regularly re-assess the vascular status.
- Manage the wound according to predominant factors.

- In the long term, prevention of arterial recurrence may depend on surgical intervention.
- Health education including advice on diet, exercise and smoking may be beneficial.

Patient involvement and compliance in ulcer management

The patient needs to be involved in the assessment, care and aftercare from the outset as this is more likely to aid compliance. Booklets and verbal information given in a patient friendly manner explaining some anatomy and physiology of the leg, why the ulcer occurred and how best to resolve the problem will enable the patient to give informed consent. The practitioner should remember that the patient has to decide if he wishes to commence and carry on with the treatment, which can take many months, so giving as much information as possible is always a positive move.

Staff education

To manage patients with leg ulcers effectively, nurses require sufficient knowledge of the underlying pathology and principles of wound management. This recommendation is supported in *The Effective Health Care Bulletin* (1997) summarises that nurses should be adequately trained in leg ulcer management and systems should be established to monitor standards of care.

As the management of leg ulcers becomes nurse led, the increase in professional responsibility brings with it new challenges which can only be met by a sound theoretical basis and knowledge. The delivery of high quality care through clinical governance should enable practitioners to ensure that the lifelong process of continuous professional development provides the means to access and learn new skills in leg ulcer management. Whilst formal courses provide the theory, access may be limited due to high cost and study time allocation.

Role of the nurse in the outpatient department

This may be the patient's first visit to a hospital for the care of their leg ulcer therefore, the role of the outpatient nurse is vital to gain an individual's trust and ensure that the lifestyle, social, physical and psychological assessment is considered with the treatment objectives. The outpatient department is an ideal venue to implement interdisciplinary teamwork into the decision on treatment and the nurse's role in leg ulcer management. Most patients enjoy facilitative learning and patient information although the nurse must be aware to consider the ethical issues of informed consent when teaching. One of the key elements of clinical governance is to ensure effective training for colleagues therefore, it is important that time and resources are allocated for teaching leg ulcer management within acute hospitals.

Patient education

The introduction of nurse led clinics creates opportunities for patient education, health promotion and more time to be spent discussing wider aspects of the problems associated with leg ulcer management. Patients with venous or arterial ulcers may require nutritional advice or supplements as the underlying pathology is not always conducive to wound healing. Extra zinc and Vitamin C may be required and in addition proteins may be depleted if exudates levels are high. It is clear that nurses have a major role in the management of patients with leg ulcers and outpatient departments can be centres of excellence where practitioners keep abreast of research and improvements in practice with the support of the tissue viability nurse and multi-disciplinary team.

Wound management/treatment options

Many leg ulcer treatments have been used on patients over the years, including topical applications of cobwebs, charcoal, marmite and rhubarb, although it is now widely accepted that the introduction of sustained graduated compression is essential for optimum healing (Eagle, 1999). Today it is well recognised that "moist wound healing" is the desirable environment for wound care. An enormous amount of work has been carried out on different dressings and nurses require a better understanding of the products.

The management of the leg ulcer wound must be part of a well thought out protocol including assessment, cleansing and measurement. Knowledge of wound care products ensures that product selection is made on a rational basis. In the absence of evident dressings should be low cost and non-adherent to avoid damage to the ulcer bed.

KEY POINTS

- 1–2% of the population has a leg ulcer at any one time.
- The cost to the NHS is estimated at £400 million per year.
- It is important to remember that a leg ulcer is a symptom of an underlying problem, not just a wound.

REFERENCES

Bosanquet N (1992) Costs of venous leg ulcers: from maintenance therapy to investment programs. *Phlebology* 290(Suppl 1): 44–46.

Browse NL, Burnand KG & Thomas ML (1988) *Diseases of the Veins: Pathology, Diagnosis and Treatment*. Edward Arnold, Baltimore.

Eagle M (1999) Compression bandaging. *Nursing Standard* 13(20): 49–56.

Laing W (1992) *Chronic Venous Diseases of the Leg*. Office of Health Economics, London.

Morgan DA (1987) Formulary of wound management products.

Morison M & Moffatt C (1994) *A Colour Guide to the Assessment and Management of Leg Ulcers*, 2nd edition. Mosby, London.

Nelson E *et al.* (1995) The management of leg ulcers. *J Wound Care* 5(2): 73–76.

Simon DA, Frank L & Williams IM (1994) Progress of arterial disease in patients with healed venous ulcers. *J Wound Care* 3(4): 179–180.

The Effective Health Care Bulletin (1997) Compression therapy for venous leg ulcers. *Publications from the NHS Centre for Reviews and Dissemination*, University of York, August 3–4.

1.10   THE DIABETIC FOOT

M. Weddell and H. Al-khaffaf

Diabetic foot problems are one of the commonest causes of admission to hospital for diabetic sufferers.

In the UK diabetic foot problems are a common complication of diabetes with prevalences of 23–42% for neuropathy, 9–23% for vascular disease and 5–7% for foot ulceration.

Diabetes is the leading cause of lower extremity amputations. A diabetic patient is 15 times more likely to have an amputation than a non-diabetic.

Most of these problems are preventable through proper care and supervision of a podiatric surgeon/nurse. These specialists can provide information on foot inspection and care, proper footwear, and early recognition and treatment of foot conditions.

St. VINCENT'S DECLARATION

In 1989 representatives of government health departments and patients' organisations from all European countries met diabetes experts in St. Vincent in Italy. They made a number of recommendations for member states aiming to improve care and reduce morbidity for diabetic people. One of the main targets was to reduce the numbers of limb amputations for diabetic gangrene by 50% in a 5-year period.

Aetiology and clinical features

Foot problems in people with diabetes are usually the result of four main factors:

1. *Peripheral neuropathy*: Damage of the sensory nerves will diminish the ability of patients to detect sensations and vibrations. As a result injuries may remain unnoticed for a lengthy period of time. Occasionally neuropathy may be painful particularly at night. Neuropathy can also damage the nerves that supply the muscles "motor neuropathy" causing muscle weakness and the development of foot deformities.

2. *Peripheral vascular disease (PVD)*: This may result in stenosis or occlusion of peripheral vessels causing intermittent claudication or critical ischaemia.
3. *Callus or deformities*: Due to peripheral neuropathy.
4. *Decreased resistance to infection*: Diabetic patients are more prone to infections and this is particularly so in patients with poorly controlled diabetes.

Diabetic feet are usually classified as neuropathic, ischaemic or neuro-ischaemic according to the predominant clinical features. Table 1.10.1 shows how to distinguish between the three types clinically (Figures 1.10.1–1.10.5).

Management

The key part in the management of foot problems in diabetics is prevention. This can be achieved by the education of patients about foot care and good diabetic control as well as regular foot inspection as part of an annual diabetic check. Such measures can help the early recognition and treatment of many of these problems. For assessment and referral pathways please see Tables 1.10.2 and 1.10.3, Figures 1.10.6 and 1.10.7.

In cases of peripheral neuropathy preventative measures is all that is required. However, if there is severe pain simple analgesia may not be adequate and antidepressants and gabapentin should be added.

If there is evidence of PVD the patient should be referred to a vascular surgeon for assessment and further management. This will be along similar lines to the management of PVD in non-diabetics (see Chapter 1.1).

Diabetic ulcers

Due to the complex aetiology of diabetic ulcers, a thorough evaluation is crucial before any treatment is instituted.

This evaluation should determine whether the ulcer is neuropathic, neuro-ischaemic or ischaemic.

An adequate description of the ulcer in terms of size, depth, appearance and location is also important, as it will help monitor the progress of treatment.

If there is evidence of infection a swab should be taken for culture and sensitivity and appropriate antibiotics should be given.

Table 1.10.1: Definition of neuropathic, neuro-ischaemic and ischaemic feet

	Neuropathic	Neuro-ischaemic	Ischaemic
Temperature	Foot is warm	Foot is warm (due to the autonomic neuropathy dilating blood vessels)	Cold
Colour	Normal/red	Pale – white/mottled red (due to dilation of vessels)	White/cyanosed depending on whether acute or chronic
Pulses	Palpable/bounding	Can be palpable/weak	Non-palpable
Pain	None usually but patient can complain of painful neuropathy	May not complain of ischaemic pain due to neuropathy	Complains of intermittent claudication on exercise "march distance"/rest pain
Ulceration	Occurs mainly on pressure areas under callus. Plantar	Occurs usually on borders of the foot	Usually occurs on borders of the foot and apex of toes
Gangrene	Due to unnoticed infection – wet gangrene travels fast	Due to poor blood supply. Dry gangrene or wet if infection is involved	Due to poor blood supply. Dry gangrene or wet if infection is involved
Skin	Dry, fissures around the heels. Heavy callus formation on pressure areas	Hair loss, fragile skin, thin dry and shiny (glassy), flaky, thickened nails, little formation of callus	Hair loss, fragile skin, thin dry and shiny (glassy), flaky, thickened nails, little formation of callus
Foot structure	Charcot deformity, prominent metatarsal heads, high arch, retracted toes, muscle wasting, anterior leg pain when walking if not masked by neuropathy	Clawed/retracted toes, prominent metatarsal heads due to atrophy of the fatty pad as well as neuropathy retraction	Clawed toes

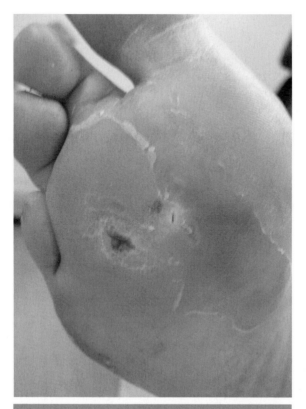

Fig. 1.10.1: Neuropathic ulceration underneath callus formation.

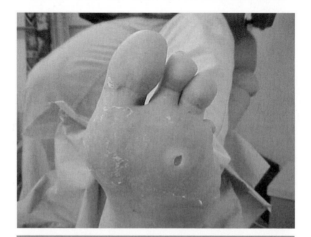

Fig. 1.10.2: Neuropathic ulceration from pressure.

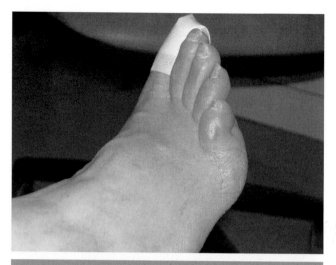

Fig. 1.10.3: Ischaemic foot.

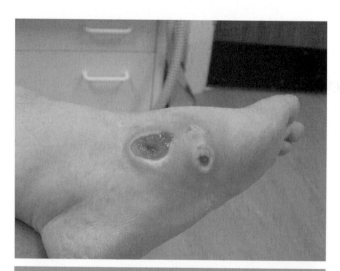

Fig. 1.10.4: Neuropathic ulceration on a foot with Charcot arthropathy.

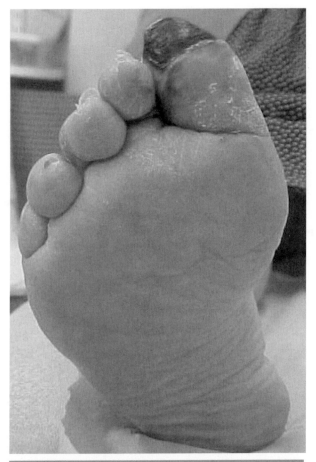

Fig. 1.10.5: Ischaemic gangrene on apex of right 1st toe.

If the ulcer is deep or chronic an X-ray of the foot should be done to exclude an underlying osteomylitis.

In the presence of critical ischaemia the patient should be referred to a vascular surgeon for further investigation and management. As in non-diabetic patients, balloon angioplasty and surgical revascularisation have been shown to reduce the rate of amputations in diabetics.

It should be acknowledged that a multi-disciplinary approach by the diabetic team, podiatrist, and the vascular team is essential for the success of treatment.

Table 1.10.2: Grading the foot for referral, follow-up and education

Vascular	Neurological using a 10 g monofilament						
	Sensory present on 10 sites	4 sites lost on same foot	4 sites lost on same foot + foot deformity	History of amputation, ulceration or charcot deformity	Non-infected ulceration	Redness, swelling, history of trauma (charcot)	Infected ulceration (see wound care guidelines)
2 Palpable pulses 1 Palpable pulse	0	1	2	3	4A	4B	5
Pulses not palpable doppler – bi phasic	1	1	2	3	4A	4B	5
Pulses not palpable doppler – mono phasic	2	2	2	3	4A	4B	5
Pulses absent with palpation and doppler	6	6	6	6	6	6	6
Black toes	6	6	6	6	6	6	6
Wound on lateral borders of foot/toes – black eschar, sloughy	6	6	6	6	6	6	6
White foot pulseless, very cold, sudden onset, very painful	7	7	7	7	7	7	7

Table 1.10.3: Care pathway according to your assessment

	Category	0	1	2	3	4A	4B 5 6 7
Primary care	Practice nurse GP Comm pod Comm nurse	12 month review		Register with pod review 3/4 months	Assess footwear. Pod review 1/2 months	Shared care between all community staff. Pressure relief	
Secondary care	Diab pod Consultant						Urgent referral to diabetic podiatrist or consultant by phone

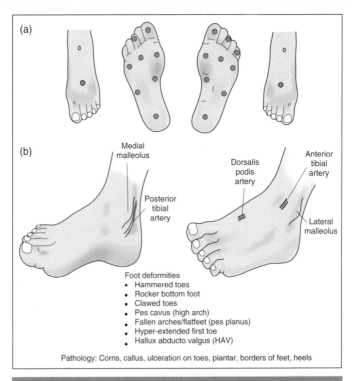

(a)

(b)

Medial malleolus

Posterior tibial artery

Dorsalis podis artery

Anterior tibial artery

Lateral malleolus

Foot deformities
• Hammered toes
• Rocker bottom foot
• Clawed toes
• Pes cavus (high arch)
• Fallen arches/flatfeet (pes planus)
• Hyper-extended first toe
• Hallux abducto valgus (HAV)

Pathology: Corns, callus, ulceration on toes, plantar, borders of feet, heels

Fig. 1.10.6: Pathways used for foot screening within podiatry. (a) ten sites for neuropathy (b) position of pulses.

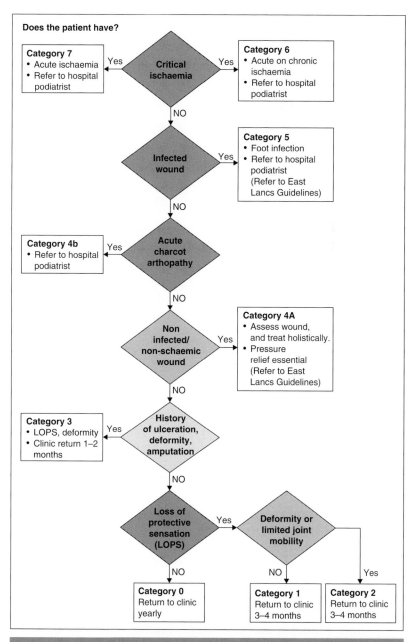

Fig. 1.10.7: Diabetic classification according to Table 1.10.3. (Taken from *Diabetes/Metabolism Research and Reviews* 2000; 16 (suppl 1): S84–S92 International consensus and practical guidelines on the management and prevention of the Diabetic Foot).

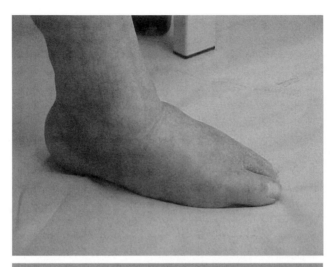

Fig. 1.10.8: A foot with a healed Charcot arthropathy that leads to deformity (collapse of medial arch) and rocker bottom foot.

Charcot arthropathy

- Usually occurs in diabetics with a duration of more than 12 years (Figure 1.10.8).
- It is associated with a mixed peripheral neuropathy and good peripheral circulation.
- Affects 1% of the diabetic population.
- Patients have a history of poor blood-sugar control.
- Often can be associated with small trauma, tripping over a stone, kerb edge.
- It has three stages: acute, bony destruction, and stabilisation stage.
  1. *Acute*:
     - Hot swollen foot usually unilateral.
     - Palpable pulses depending on swelling, can be bounding.
     - Painless but can have an unremitting ache (differential diagnosis: cellulitis, septic arthritis, gout, DVT, osteomyelitis).
     - X-ray will appear normal, bone scan will show changes in the bone. Refer to secondary care – Diabetes Team.
     - Treatment: with Biphosphate infusion to reduce osteoclast activity. Immobilisation and non-weight bearing until swelling and temperature have subsided.
  2. *Bony destruction*: X-ray shows fragmentation and fractures and new bone formation, subluxation and dislocation. Treatment is by immobilisation until bony destruction is not seen on X-ray.
  3. *Stabilisation*: The foot is no longer warm and red but may still be swollen. X-ray will show healing and remodelling.

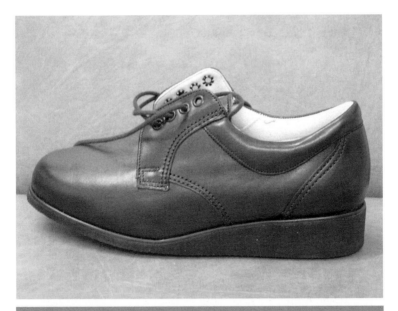

Fig. 1.10.9: Surgical appliance stock shoe.

Treatment: Total contact orthosis and footwear to accommodate any deformities. Gradually increasing walk and alternating between footwear and walker. Monitoring of foot on a regular basis is essential. Patient may need surgery if foot is unstable.

- All diabetic patients that have undergone minor or major amputation or have had foot ulceration should be assessed for footwear and total contact insoles (Figure 1.10.9)

REFERENCES

Diabetes/Metabolism Research and Reviews (2000): 16 (suppl 1): S84–S92. International consensus and practical guidelines on the management and prevention of the Diabetic Foot).

Edmonds M & Foster A (2000) *Managing the Diabetic Foot*. Blackwell Science, Oxford.

Katsilambros N, Tentoluris N, Tsapogas P & Dounis E (2003) *Atlas of the Diabetic Foot*. John Wiley & Sons, Chichester, England.

The charcot foot in diabetes "six key points": Gregory et al. June. Published by American Academy of Family Physicians.

FURTHER READING

Scottish Intercollegiate Guidelines Network (2001) *Management of Diabetes*. SIGN Publication No. 55.

http://www.sign.ac.uk/guidelines/fulltext/55/

1.11   MESENTERIC ISCHAEMIA

H. Al-Khaffaf

Ischaemic bowel disease can be either acute or chronic.

ACUTE MESENTERIC ISCHAEMIA

- Is a rare condition caused by occlusion of either the superior mesenteric artery or vein.
- In the majority of cases the occlusion is embolic, with emboli originating from either the heart or an atherosclerotic aorta. Acute thrombosis of an atheromatous mesenteric artery accounts for about 25% of cases while acute mesenteric venous thrombosis is extremely rare.

Clinical features

- Acute abdominal pain of variable severity, nature and location.
- The pain is usually out of proportion to physical findings in early stages.
- Rapid and forceful bowel evacuation.
- Atrial fibrillation or a recent history of myocardial infarction.
- Symptoms of chronic bowel ischaemia may be present in cases of arterial thrombosis.
- Abdominal distension is a late feature and is often the first sign of impending bowel infarction.
- Markedly raised white cell count with metabolic acidosis.

Diagnosis

- Early identification requires a high index of suspicion.
- Abdominal X-ray may be normal early in the disease process. However, late films may show dilated small bowel and "thumb printing" due to mucosal oedema.
- Angiography may confirm the diagnosis.

Management

Once the diagnosis is suspected, aggressive resuscitation and urgent laparotomy are required. If the bowel is still viable, embolectomy or bypass surgery can be performed to improve blood flow. Non-viable bowel should be resected, however, because the diagnosis is often delayed resection may be of no benefit due to extensive ischaemia and bowel infarction. Mortality is usually high and has been reported to be 50–90%.

CHRONIC MESENTERIC ISCHAEMIA

Chronic mesenteric ischaemia (CMI) is an uncommon condition caused by atherosclerotic narrowing of the main mesenteric arteries. Due to the good collateral circulation, symptoms will only develop when the blood supply to the gut is severely compromised.

Clinical features

- Colicky, epigastric pain occurring 30–60 min after eating (post-brandial).
- Food fear, with severe weight loss and cachexia.
- On examination an abdominal bruit may be heard.

Diagnosis

- Due to the associated marked weight loss it is essential to exclude abdominal malignancies.
- Duplex scan can accurately identify high-grade stenosis in the superior mesenteric artery and the coeliac axis, and may be used as an early non-invasive screening procedure for patients with symptoms suggestive of CMI.
- Selective angiography is essential to confirm the diagnosis of CMI as well as aid in planning revascularisation. It should include a lateral view of the aorta and the origins of the main vessels.

Treatment

Treatment is by surgical reconstruction of one or more of the mesenteric arteries. Vascular reconstructive techniques include bypass, endarterectomy and reimplantation. Balloon angioplasty with or without stenting is an acceptable alternative in patients who are not fit for surgery although recurrence is a major concern.

REFERENCE

http://emedicine.com/EMERG/topic311.htm

1.12   VARICOSE VEINS

M.A. Rahi

Anatomy

The venous system of the legs comprises a superficial system in the skin and subcutaneous fat, a deep system beneath the fascia and in leg muscles, and the perforator veins which connect the two systems.

The superficial system is a venous network with prominent long and short saphenous veins as shown in Figure 1.12.1.

Patho-physiology

Blood is returned from the legs against gravity by the pumping action of the calf muscles and to a lesser extent the foot and thigh muscles. Superficial veins

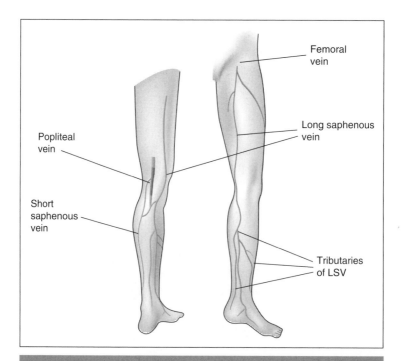

Fig. 1.12.1: Anatomy of superficial veins in the lower limbs.

collect blood from the superficial tissues, and when the deep muscles relax, this blood enters the deep system via the perforating veins (Figure 1.12.2).

Superficial, deep and perforating veins have several venous valves which guard and maintain the correct direction of the flow of blood, i.e. flow from superficial into the deep veins via the perforating veins as shown.

Incompetence of the venous valves permits reflux and so the veins dilate, become tortuous and varicose as illustrated in Figure 1.12.3.

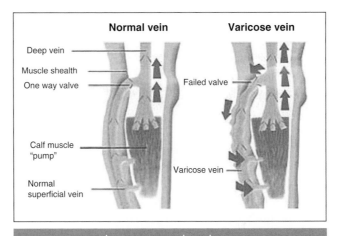

Fig. 1.12.2: Flow in normal and varicose veins.

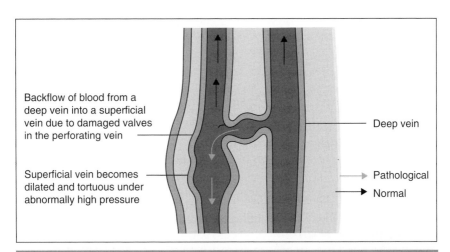

Fig. 1.12.3: Haemodynamic changes in varicose veins.

Assessment in outpatient clinic

There are three important questions which need to be considered on assessment of patients who are referred by the general practitioner (GP) with varicose veins.

- Are the symptoms due to varicose veins?
- Is there deep venous pathology?
- Is there arterial disease?

History

Patients who present with pain and discomfort in their legs may have other conditions. It is important to assess the symptoms due to varicose veins and to exclude the symptoms due to orthopaedic, neurological and arterial causes. Past history of deep venous thrombus (DVT) and leg surgery should be noted.

Examination

- *General physical*: Body weight, blood pressure (BP), pulse, urinalysis.
- *Abdominal examination*: To exclude abdominal and pelvic pathology.
- *Musculo-skeletal*: To examine lower back, hips and knees.
- *Peripheral pulses*: To palpate pulses and do ankle-brachial pressure indices.

Leg examination for varicose veins on standing.

Investigations

Varicose veins are investigated by following tests, only if treatment is indicated.

Hand-held Doppler examination

Hand-held Doppler examination is a useful test to confirm the presence of reflux signal due to valve failure at sapheno-femoral junction (in groin) and possibly at sapheno–popliteal junction (behind the knee).

Colour duplex scan

Patients who had DVT, previous varicose vein surgery and suspected of having short saphenous and deep venous incompetence should undergo duplex examination for further assessment in vascular laboratory (Figure 1.12.4).

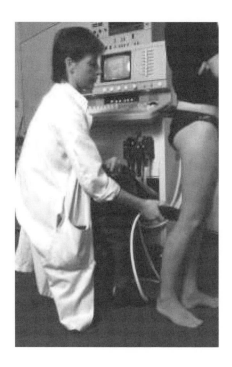

Fig. 1.12.4: Duplex scan examination of varicose veins.

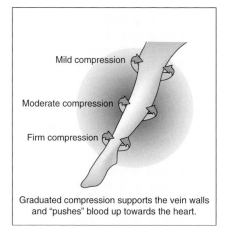

Mild compression

Moderate compression

Firm compression

Graduated compression supports the vein walls and "pushes" blood up towards the heart.

Fig. 1.12.5: Mechanism of graduated compression stockings.

Treatment options of varicose veins

Depends on the patient and their symptoms. The treatment options are as follows:

- No intervention if quality of life is not affected.
- Graduated compression stockings for high-risk patients (Figure 1.12.5).

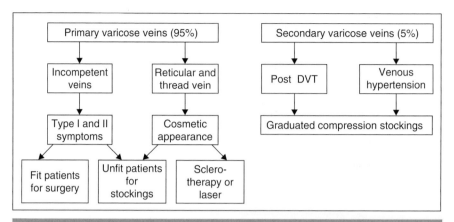

Fig. 1.12.6: Management plan of varicose veins.

- Injection sclerotherapy for reticular veins.
- Laser treatment for thread veins.
- Surgery for symptomatic patients who are fit (see Chapter 5.3).

Management plan

The management plan is shown in Figure 1.12.6.

REFERENCES

Callam MJ (1994) Epidemiology of varicose veins. *Br J Surg* 81: 167–173.

Campbell WB, Niblett PG, Ridler BMF, Peters AS & Thompson JF (1997) Hand-held Doppler as a screening test in primary varicose veins. *Br J Surg* 84: 1541–1543.

Darke SG, Vetrivel S, Foy DMA, Smith S & Baker S (1997) A comparison of duplex scanning and continuous wave Doppler in the assessment of primary and uncomplicated varicose veins. *Eur J Vasc Endovasc Surg* 14: 457–461.

Lees TA & Holdsworth JD (1995) Assessment and treatment of varicose veins in the Northern Region. *Phleboloby* 10: 56–61.

Mercer KG, Scott DJA & Berridge DC (1998) Preoperative duplex imaging is required before all operations for primary varicose veins. *Br J Surg* 85: 1495–1497.

1.13   DEEP VEIN THROMBOSIS

H. Al-Khaffaf

- Formation of clots in the deep vein is a common and potentially serious condition.
- The true incidence of deep vein thrombosis (DVT) is unknown. However, it is estimated that about one in 2000 people in the UK develops a DVT each year.
- Its most important acute complication, pulmonary embolism is highly preventable. It accounts for 3% of hospital inpatients deaths.
- About 80% of DVTs dissolve spontaneously without treatment.
- The most common site for DVT is the calf veins. However, only about 20% of these patients will have proximal propagation of thrombus.
- Proximal DVT is associated with a 10% risk of pulmonary embolism.
- Recently there has been a lot of media publicity about DVT in air passengers. It has been dubbed "economy class syndrome" because of its association with cramped conditions in cheaper airline seats.

Causes

In 1856, Virchow identified three major factors that may initiate DVT (Table 1.13.1). These are changes of vessel wall, blood flow stasis and increased coagulability of blood.

Table 1.13.1: Patients at risk of venous thromboembolism

Causes	Examples
Change of vessel wall	Femoral vein damage in total hip replacement
Blood flow stasis	
More time for clotting	Sitting still "Long hall flight"
Small thrombi not washed away	Limb paralysis
Viscosity increased	Heart failure
	Varicose veins
Coagulability	
Increase in tissue factor	Surgery
Presence of activating factors	Cancer
Decrease in coagulation inhibitors	Inherited AT III deficiency

Risk factors

People at risk of getting a DVT:

- Age: People over 40 are at a higher risk.
- Patients with a previous history of venous thrombosis.
- Obesity.
- Thrombophilia: The tendency to form blood clot can increase due to several inherited conditions like antithrombin III deficiency, protein C deficiency, protein S deficiency and antiphospholipid antibody.
- Prolonged bed rest (immobility).
- Patients with varicose veins.
- Major injuries or paralysis.
- Surgery, especially if it lasts more than 30 min, or involves the leg joints or pelvis.
- Cancer and its treatments, which can cause the blood to clot more easily.
- Infection.
- Long-distance travel, because of prolonged immobility. It is unclear whether or not air travel is more risky than other long journeys, e.g. by car or coach.
- Pregnancy and childbirth – related to hormone changes that make the blood clot more easily and because the foetus puts added pressure on the veins of the pelvis. There is also risk of injury to veins during delivery or a caesarean. The risk is at its highest just after childbirth.
- Taking a contraceptive pill that contains oestrogen. Most modern pills contain a low dose, which increases the risk by an amount, i.e. acceptable for most women.
- Hormone replacement therapy (HRT). For many women, the benefits outweigh the increase in risk.
- Other circulation or heart problems.

Clinical features

- Many of the patients have no symptoms (silent DVT). In fact pulmonary embolism may be the primary presentation.
- Some patients may experience a dull aching pain in the calf or thigh which may be worse on walking or standing.
- There may be swelling with redness of the legs and some patients may have a low-grade fever.
- On examination, apart from the swelling, there may be tenderness in the calf and the skin is warm to touch. Bluish discolouration of the skin may be present.
- Homan's sign, pain on dorsiflexion of the foot may be positive but is not reliable.

Diagnosis

- As the symptoms of DVT are non-specific clinical diagnosis is often unreliable. However, a high index of suspicion is recommended in high-risk patients.
- A clinical diagnosis must be confirmed with an objective test as treatment is not without risk.
- Duplex scan is a highly reliable non-invasive test and has replaced venography which is considered to be the "gold standard". In modern practice venography is only considered if the result of Duplex scan is inconclusive.
- The levels of D-dimers (a fibrin degradation product that can be assayed in plasma) is raised in the presence of a recent thrombus. A negative result almost excludes DVT and it is now routinely used if DVT is suspected before a decision to proceed with ultrasound or venography is made.

Prevention

- Several studies have shown that the incidence of DVT can be significantly reduced by the appropriate use of prophylaxis in high-risk patients.
- Protocols for prophylaxis are based on risk assessment and vary from hospital to hospital.
- The common practice in hospital patients is to give a low-molecular weight heparin (LMWH) subcutaneously from the day of admission till the day of discharge.
- Prophylaxis should also include early mobilisation and graduated compression stockings. Intermittent pneumatic compression, e.g. flowtron boots is also recommended.

Treatment

- The main aim of the treatment is the prevention of pulmonary embolism.
- Treatment is by anticoagulation. Traditionally, 5000 u of unfractionated heparin are given intravenously (i.v.) as a bolus dose followed by continuous i.v. infusion. However, over the past few years therapeutic doses of LMWH have been increasingly used subcutaneously instead of fractionated heparin.
- Oral anticoagulation with warfarin should then be commenced and continued for 3–6 months.
- Compression hosiery and leg elevation should be advised to prevent long-term complications.
- The role of thrombolysis and surgical thrombectomy is not clear but may be considered in cases of extensive proximal DVT.
- Treatment of calf veins DVT is controversial.

Complications

Complications of DVT are of following two types:

1. Acute
   - The most important acute complication is pulmonary embolism. However, DVT of the legs can be demonstrated only in 30–40% of patients with pulmonary embolism.
   - DVT can cause severe venous obstruction leading to venous gangrene.
2. Chronic
   - The only chronic complication is chronic deep vein incompetence (also known as post-phlebitic syndrome), which may lead to leg swelling, secondary varisosity and ulceration.

REFERENCES

Belcaro G, Nicolaides AN & Veller M (1995). *Venous Disorders*. WB Saunders, London.
http://www.umassmed.edu/outcomes/dvt/Chapt1-frameset.html

1.14 MANAGING LYMPHOEDEMA: A CLINIC APPROACH

J.C. Whitaker

Lymphoedema is a progressive chronic swelling of the limbs and the body that occurs as a result of an inadequate compromised lymphatic system.

The most common form is in a limb, but it can affect any part of the body.

At present there are no accurate figures of the number of people with lymphoedema, although it has been estimated that 144 per 100,000 are affected. (Casley-Smith, 1997). Predominantly in the literature breast cancer related swelling is the most quoted, and this equates to an incidence and prevalence following diagnosis and treatment of 25–28% occurrence (Logan, 1995; Kissen *et al.*, 1996).

Lymphoedema is classified as either primary or secondary:

- *Primary lymphoedema*: Is due to underdevelopment of the lymphatic system. Three different types have been recognised.
  - *Congenital lymphoedema (Milory's disease)*: Present at or within a year of birth. It is more common in males and more likely to be bilateral and involve the whole leg.
  - *Lymphoedema praecox*: Appears during puberty and is the most common form of primary lymphoedema. It is more common in females and more likely to be unilateral and only extends to the knee.
  - *Lymphoedema tarda*: Appears later in life, i.e. from 30 to 40 onwards. It is important that when lymphoedema develops for the first time in later life, an underlying malignancy is excluded.
- *Secondary lymphoedema*: Occurs when the lymphatic system becomes impaired following surgery and/or radiotherapy (as in cancer treatment), or also as a result of infection, severe injury, burns or trauma.

Diagnosis

Very often the diagnosis is easy and can be established from the history and clinical examination. Occasionally, however, it can be difficult and investigations are required to exclude other causes of limb swelling.

The best diagnostic test for lymphoedema is lymphoscintigraphy.

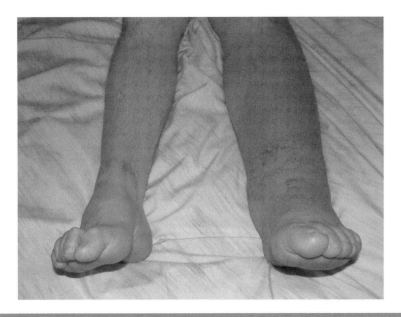

Fig. 1.14.1: Primary lymphoedema with cellulitis.

Management

Lymphoedema is a chronic ongoing condition. Although it can never be cured, it can be greatly improved.

The implementation of treatment aims to control and reduce the swelling, prevent progression of lymphoedema, reverse complications and provide patients with an ongoing maintenance plan of care to improve patient's over-all quality of life.

Effective management has been shown to significantly reduce the incidence of cellulitis (acute infection) and the possible need for hospital admission (Mortimer, 1995; Todd, 1999), both of which are common problems encountered with lymphoedema.

By improving health and independence, effective lymphoedema management can minimise the demands of increasing immobility and discomfort that would otherwise be made on the health services.

This development addresses the recommendation within the Calman-Hine report that: "nursing services must be structured to ensure access to specialist nurses with specialist skills, e.g. lymphoedema."

LYMPHOEDEMA CLINICS

Key-worker role within the clinic

Adequate provision will need to be made to offer existing and newly diagnosed patients with lymphoedema a maintenance service.

Nurses and/or physiotherapists within the Medical and Surgical Departments who have completed a training course at key-worker level will run the clinic. This will enable them to offer a maintenance service. A key-worker is educated and trained to offer the following:

- Comprehensive assessment of patients with lymphoedema unique to their needs. Measurable tools will be included within the assessment process to monitor clinical effectiveness and contribute to ongoing audit of the service. These will include 4 cm cylindrical limb volume measurements, skin and subcutaneous tissue score, pain and psychological visual analogue scales (VAS), distribution of swelling, function and movement. Screening tools for onward referral to the lymphoedema specialist for intensive treatment are also implemented.
- The maintenance service will enable the nurse/physiotherapist to offer the patient advice and ongoing support on a self-care programme consisting of compression hosiery, exercise, skin care and simple lymphatic drainage (SLD).
- Due to the chronic nature of lymphoedema a key-worker is in a position to monitor long-term care and refer onwards to the appropriate specialist as necessary.
- They will also be able to offer fellow colleagues and patients basic information, education and advice within their own clinical setting.
- The key-worker has not undertaken specialist treatment interventions, therefore is not in a position to offer intensive treatment sessions, e.g. manual lymphatic drainage (MLD) and multi-layer lymphoedema bandaging (MLLB). Referral to a lymphoedema specialist is essential if the treatment is required.
- To be pro-active in the audit of the lymphoedema service.
- The clinic provides a structured set-up to enable the key-worker access to a multi-professional team to meet the individual needs of the patient.

To ensure practitioners are equipped with appropriate knowledge and skills to comprehensively assess and meet the individual needs of the patients under their care, the following provision for education needs careful consideration.

Education

- An accredited course which will provide comprehensive assessment skills unique to lymphoedema management at maintenance level; detailed physiological function of the lymphatic system; skills to implement the four

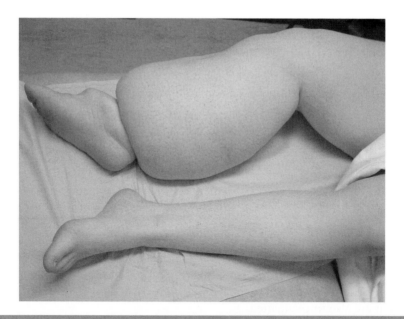

Fig. 1.14.2: Secondary lymphoedema following excision of lymph nodes from the right groin.

cornerstones of treatment – skin care, hosiery, SLD and exercise, is required. Monitoring of treatment response and long-term progress for mild and uncomplicated lymphoedema. Address the management of patients with advancing disease and adapt appropriate treatments.

- An agreeable period of clinical supervision between newly qualified key-worker and lymphoedema clinical nurse specialist (CNS).

Other areas to consider

- Referral pathways.
- Audit and research.
- Administration.
- Equipment.
- BUDGET!

Patient intervention

Thorough assessment is critical to meet the needs of the patient. Important contextual factors and ideological concerns must be taken into account to ensure the patient suffering with this condition is managed holistically.

The involvement of the multi-disciplinary team at an early stage must be recognised and referred to as appropriate.

When assessing a patient, the following should be taken into consideration:

- Biographical details,
- Other professionals involved in the care,
- Previous medical/surgical history,
- Relevant health problems,
- Cancer status (if appropriate),
- Current medication and allergies,
- History and development of oedema,
- Detailed history of acute inflammatory episode (AIE),
- Lifestyle and social factors,
- Pain and sensation scores,
- Psychosocial/logical impact of oedema,
- Function and movement,
- Site and distribution of oedema,
- Skin and subcutaneous tissue state.

When this thorough assessment has been completed, only then can a realistic diagnosis be made. Following this, the formulation of a detailed treatment plan of action should be drawn up.

TREATMENT PLAN – POSSIBLE CONSIDERATIONS
Surgery

Surgical intervention to manage lymphoedema has been practiced for many years, however, despite many attempts to perfect techniques to improve limb function and reduce tissue, <10% of all patients benefit from surgery (Carrell & Burnard, 2000). Historically, surgical techniques, such as Charles, Thompson's and Homan's operation/procedures were used, again with little benefit. The main aim of these three techniques was de-bulking the tissue to achieve a reduction. More recently, techniques using anastomosis of the lymphatic and venous structures to encourage flow have been used. Unfortunately, long-term results for these patients have proved to be unsuccessful.

Non-surgical approach

This approach consists of MLD, compression bandaging, exercise therapy and patient education regarding skin care.

The rational and techniques of these treatments are explained below based on an information leaflet given to the patients in the clinics.

Why take care of your skin?

Lymphoedema is an excess of water, large proteins and waste material, which has accumulated in the tissues. This is an ideal environment for bacteria to manifest. In some cases, the lymph nodes may have been removed, therefore, the local immune system may be compromised in the swollen area. All of these factors contribute to the increased risk of developing an AIE (cellulitis). Taking care of your skin, minimises the increased risk of infection, which often accompanies lymphatic disorders.

How to take care of your skin

Scrupulous hygiene techniques performed to the swollen area, daily, will help to preserve the health of the skin. A thorough drying technique to the area should be adopted to prevent breakdown of the skin. By choosing an unperfumed, simple moisturiser and applying it daily will help keep the skin hydrated and supple, thus preventing dryness and cracks developing. A lanolin-free cream available from your general practitioner (GP) called DIPROBASE will help with this maintenance.

Why exercise?

It is important to encourage the lymphatic system to perform its function. By performing the exercises in this leaflet, we aim to achieve the following:

- To increase the uptake of fluid by the lymphatics.
- To encourage the deep (large vessels) lymphatics to pump better.
- To mobilise the joints making the muscles pump fluid into the lymphatics.
- To strengthen the muscles of the limb to help avoid any muscle wastage often seen in long-standing lymphoedema.
- To maintain and improve the function and dexterity of the limb.

It is recommended that these exercises are done as well as the normal daily use of the limb. Best results will be achieved when wearing your prescribed compression garment whilst exercising.

Swimming is a good all round exercise, as any movement in the water supports your swollen limb.

When to AVOID exercising?

- In the presence of an acute infection, inflammation, such as cellulitis, erysipelas, flu or active tuberculosis.
- In the presence of an acute injury to the affected area.

What are compression garments/hosiery?

Compression garments or hosiery, are elasticated garments, which are worn over a swollen limb. For arm swelling a sleeve is worn and for leg swelling a stocking is worn. Several sizes, styles and colours are available for both arm and leg oedema, to achieve maximum benefit.

Why wear compression garments/hosiery?

Wearing compression garments daily over your swollen limb will help to control and contain the oedema. It will also improve the shape and size of your limb. Compression aims to reduce new lymph formation and enhance lymph drainage by improving muscle pump efficiency. It may be necessary in some cases to layer the garments to increase the level of support given.

How to apply your garment

It is advisable to wear rubber gloves to aid application making it much easier to grip and adjust the garment. Compression garments are tight, therefore quite difficult to apply. If you have problems, contact your lymphoedema therapist as they may have some aids, which may ease application.

How to care for your garment

You will be supplied with two sleeves from your lymphoedema therapist, one to wear and one to wash. All hosiery can be hand washed or machine washed at 40°C or less. Never dry your garment over direct heat or in a tumble dryer, as this will perish the elastic in your garment.

What is simple lymphatic drainage?

Simple Lymphatic Drainage is based on the principles of MLD. It involves the use of simple hand movements and is designed to be easily accessible for patients, relatives and carers. It is used daily within a lymphoedema treatment programme, when one is managing their own care.

Why perform simple lymphatic drainage?

To provide a technique of self-massage which provides a manual drainage route to relieve tissue congestion, which can be performed independently.

This is achieved by:

- Incorporating simplified hand movements in a set sequence, which work across the lymphatic watersheds towards the functioning lymphatics.
- Treatment is mainly to the neck and trunk area, although the limb may be treated. This depends on the needs and abilities of the individual, and the condition of the limb.
- No oils or creams are used.
- Best results are often achieved when this technique is performed whilst wearing your compression garment.

When to avoid SLD:

- In the presence of acute infection, inflammation, such as cellulitis, erysipelas, flu or active tuberculosis.
- Acute thrombosis, e.g. deep vein thrombosis (DVT) (BLS, 1999).

Manual lymphatic drainage (MLD)

This is a specialised form of massage performed by a therapist, designed to drain oedematous tissue by stimulating the lymph system. It is always performed proximal to the oedema. It aims to drain lymph from an affected area to a non-affected area and also is known to help breakdown fibrotic tissue. MLD is reported to be beneficial for other health problems. The therapist should hold a recognised certificate in MLD prior to treating patients.

Multi-layer lymphoedema bandaging (MLLB)

The application of several layers of undercast padding, varying densities of foam and short-stretch bandages are use to reshape and reduce the volume of the limb. It works well on breaking down hard fibrosis and assists the re-absorption of large proteins collected in the tissue space. It is effective in reversing skin changes, such as hyperkeritosis and lymphorrhoea. Applied daily from 1 to 3 weeks or more, MLLB is a very intensive approach to management and is usually only done on patients with complicated severe lymphoedema. The therapist, prior to application, requires specific training.

LIMB VOLUME MEASUREMENT LEG
Equipment

- Examination couch.
- Foot block.
- Ruler.
- Felt-tip washable ink pen.
- Skin wipes (not alcohol wipes).
- Pre-tension tape measure.
- Volume measurement chart.
- Programmable calculator.

Process

- Remove footwear and compression garments.
- Sit the patient on the examination couch in an upright position with legs out stretched. Adjust the height of the couch to the therapists' requirement.

- Place the foot block under the heal and up against the sole of the foot, so it sits at right angles.
- Make a start point mark on the leg with the felt-tip pen, 2 cm above the malleolous. If possible use the non-swollen leg to determine this measurement. Document it on the measurement sheet as the start point for any subsequent measurements. Use the felt pen to mark the skin.
- Using the felt pen and ruler, mark every 4 cm up the limb from the start point until you reach the top of the leg. Document the number of points marked.
- Place the tape measure *below* the first mark and record the circumference. Ensure the tape lies flat across the limb and it is level around the leg.
- Repeat this process up the limb and repeat on both sides, document each individual measurement on the chart.
- Enter the circumference measurements for both legs into the programmable calculator. To calculate the limb volume different (excess) in millilitres and per cent, and volume loss and gain. Record these on the measurement chart.
- Measure the foot by placing the tape around the dorsum/sole of the foot at mid-tarsal point. This measurement is not included in the calculation process.
- Once the measurements are completed, remove the marks with the skin wipes provided.
- Segmental comparisons of the limbs can be made by using the original measurements taken. These can be documented on the limb volume measurement chart.
- Always measure the full limb even if the oedema is only present in part of it.

REFERENCES

Carrell T & Burnard K (2000) Surgery and lymphoedema. In: Twycross R, Jenns K & Todd J (eds). *Lymphoedema*, 1st Edition. Radcliffe Medical Press Ltd, Oxford; pp. 285–292.

Casley-Smith JR (1997) *Modern Treatment for Lymphoedema*, 5th Edition. Terrance Printing, Adelaide.

Kissen MW, Querci G, Easton D & Westburg G (1996) Risk of lymphoedema following the treatment of breast cancer. *Br J Surg* 73: 580–584.

Logan V (1995) Incidence and prevalence of lymphoedema: a literature review. *J Clin Nurs* 4: 213–219.

Mortimer P (1995) Managing lymphoedema. *Clin Exp Dermatol* 20: 98–106.

Todd JE (1999) A study of two lymphoedema clinics. *Physiotherapy* 85(2): 65–75.

VASCULAR EMERGENCIES

All vascular emergencies are life threatening and the mortality is extremely high if the conditions are not diagnosed and treated speedily. Early diagnosis is essential and urgent operative management can prevent a serious adverse outcome.

Life-threatening emergencies: They can be divided into three main groups on presentation to hospital in accident and emergency unit.

2.1   RUPTURED ABDOMINAL AORTIC ANEURYSM

M.A. Rahi

Rupture and leaking of abdominal aortic aneurysm is one of the most dangerous events in vascular surgery. Half of the patients never make their journey to hospital and die in the community. Of the other half, who arrive in hospital and are considered suitable for surgical repair, only 50% survive.

DEFINITION

Aortic aneurysm is permanent localised dilatation of 3 cm and above.

AETIOLOGY

The aneurysmal aortic wall is characterised by reduction of elastin and smooth muscle cells in aortic media layer with compensatory expansion of collagenous adventitial layer with atherosclerotic degeneration of the intimal layer of aorta. These changes result in weakness of aortic wall with the consequences of tear and rupture.

RISK FACTORS

- Age >60 years.
- Hypertension.
- Sex: four times more common in males.
- Diabetes.
- Hereditary.
- Smoking.
- Hyperlipaedemia.
- Ischaemic heart disease.

PRESENTATION IN ACCIDENT AND EMERGENCY

Leaking or rupture abdominal aortic or thoracic aneurysm is usually present with one of the following symptoms:

- Sudden back pain.
- Acute abdominal pain.

- Collapse and shock.
- Sudden, severe chest pain.
- Acute lower limb ischaemia.

DIFFERENTIAL DIAGNOSIS

- Myocardial infarction (MI).
- Perforated ulcer.
- Renal or ureteric colic.
- Acute pancreatitis.
- Acute cholecystitis.
- Bowel obstruction.

CLINICAL DIAGNOSIS

The presence of a palpable and tender abdominal aorta makes a reliable clinical diagnosis in about 50% of the patients. General physical, cardio-respiratory and examination of peripheral pulses is mandatory.

INVESTIGATIONS

- Palpable, tender abdominal aortic aneurysm only requires full blood count (FBC), urea and electrolytes (U/E) and cross-match.
- Abdominal ultrasound is required only if unsure of diagnosis on clinical examination.
- Spiral computerised tomography (CT) scan is needed only for stable patients or suspected thoracic aortic aneurysm (Figure 2.1.1).

MANAGEMENT IN ACCIDENT AND EMERGENCY

Outcome of the patient depends on successful initial resuscitation by the medical and nursing team, and the important steps are outlined as follows:

- Full active resuscitation.
- Size 10–12 venflon in each arm.
- High flow oxygen 10–15 l/min.
- Inspiration/ventilation (I/V) crystalloid and colloid to keep blood pressure (BP) at 90 mmHg only.
- Call for immediate senior help.
- FBC, U/E and 10 units cross-match.

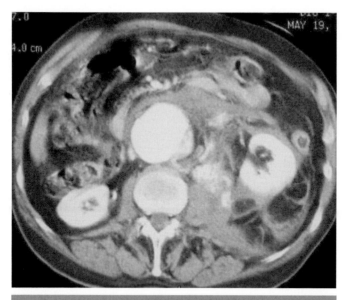

Fig. 2.1.1: CT scan of a ruptured aortic aneurysm.

- Electrocardiogram (ECG) to exclude MI.
- Catheterisation for urine output monitoring.
- Inform immediately to surgical registrar and vascular surgeon on call.
- Notify theatre.
- Speak to family of life-threatening condition.
- Old clinical notes are essential and informative.

DECISION FOR SURGERY

The final decision regarding operation is made by the consultant vascular surgeon on call after careful consideration of the following factors:

- How successful is the initial resuscitation?
- How is the patient's general medical fitness?
- What are the wishes of patient and full informed consent?
- What are the desires of the family?

OPERATIVE SURGICAL OPTIONS

Open aortic aneurysm graft repair surgery

This has been the standard treatment for over 50 years and is well established. Mortality is still 40–70% with this approach.

Emergency endo-vascular aortic aneurysm repair surgery

Emergency endo-vascular aortic aneurysm repair surgery (EVAR) has been used to repair ruptured aneurysms for nearly 10 years and the results are encouraging. The reported mortality is only 15–22%. This technique is available only in a few vascular centres at present and has a great potential for saving lives of patients.

PROGNOSIS

- 40–70% mortality even with successful open aortic aneurysm repair.
- 15–22% mortality with EVAR (if facilities are available).
- 95% mortality with single organ failure on presentation.
- 100% mortality if three criteria are present, i.e. cardiac arrest, (Glasgow Coma Scale (GCS) < 15, Hb < 6), ECG changes and renal failure.

2.2   ACUTE LIMB ISCHAEMIA

M.A. Rahi

Acute ischaemia of the leg is most common in elderly people and usually due to atherosclerosis and thrombo-embolism. Upper limb acute ischaemia is much less common and usually due to embolism and trauma. Diagnosis is often delayed in its early reversible stage.

DEFINITION

Sudden deterioration in arterial supply resulting in chest pain and/or other features of severe ischaemia of less than 2 weeks duration.

CLASSIFICATION

Acute limb ischaemia can be classified into three categories:

Category	Description	Motor loss	Sensory loss	Doppler
Viable	Not immediately threatened	No	No	Audible
Threatened	Salvageable if immediately Rx	Partial	Partial	Inaudible
Irreversible	Primary amputation	Complete	Complete	Inaudible

AETIOLOGY

Acute limb ischaemia may be due to closure of a native artery or graft. Arterial occlusion is commonly due to thrombosis or embolus. The causes for upper and lower limb ischaemia are as follows:

Embolism	Thrombosis	Others
Atrial fibrillation	Atherosclorosis	Trauma (including iatrogenic)
Recent MI	Proximal aneurysm	Dissection
Cardiac vegetations	Graft occlusion	External compression

PRESENTATION

The severity of ischaemia at presentation is variable but early diagnosis and prompt intervention determines the outcome.

Classical ischaemic limb has six "P"s

- Pain: sudden and severe.
- Pallor: white or commonly mottled.
- Pulses: loss of pulse is definite criteria.
- Paraesthesia: reduce sensations is usual.
- Paralysis: failure of dorsiflexion is not a good sign.
- Perishing cold limb is usual complaint but extent is variable.

DIFFERENTIAL DIAGNOSIS

Nerve trauma, spinal disease and stroke can be differentiated from the acute limb ischaemia, as peripheral pulses are present in all these conditions.

DIAGNOSIS

- Symptoms and signs of six "P"s.
- Absence of pulses is an absolute criterion.
- Cardiac examination to exclude cardiac source of embolus.
- Abdominal examination to diagnose aortic aneurysm.
- Lower limb examination to exclude femoral or popliteal aneurysms.

INVESTIGATIONS

- FBC, U/E, clotting and group/save.
- ECG to diagnose recent MI and atrial fibrillation (AF).
- Ankle/brachial pressure index measurement.
- Hand held Doppler examination.
- Duplex scan and angiography is informative (Figure 2.2.1).

INITIAL MANAGEMENT

These patients are in very poor clinical condition and have high mortality rate due to associated cardiovascular disease.

- Immediate oxygen to correct hypoxia.
- I/V access to correct dehydration.
- Early pain relieve by giving intravenous (i.v.) analgesia.
- ECG to diagnose AF and MI and treat accordingly.
- Inform the vascular team on call immediately.

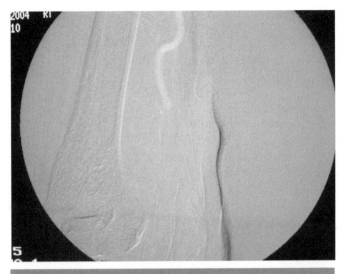

Fig. 2.2.1: An angiogram of an embolus of the right brachial artery.

- Heparin of 5000 i.u. as a bolus i.v.
- Followed by 1000 i.u. of heparin per hour i.v. as an infusion.
- Inform theatre according to operative management plan.

SURGICAL INTERVENTION

After successful initial management, further clinical assessment of the severity of limb ischaemia, dictates plan as follows:

1. Irreversible ischaemia (fixed skin staining and tense muscles): amputation.
2. Moderate ischaemia (dusky leg and mild anaesthesia): angiogram.
3. Severe ischaemia (white paralysed leg): surgical revascularisation.

REVASCULARISATION

- Surgical embolectomy when embolism is the cause (see Chapter 5.3).
- Thrombolysis when thrombosis is the cause and there is no contraindication.
- Surgical bypass graft surgery when required and indicated.

PROGNOSIS

Only 60–70% of patients admitted with an acutely ischaemic leg leave hospital with an intact limb. The 30-day mortality rate is 15–30% and 15% of survivors undergo an amputation.

2.3 VASCULAR TRAUMA

M.A. Rahi

The incidence of vascular trauma differs from centre to centre. In Europe the trauma centres report a 5–8% incidence as compared to 35% in USA.

Vascular injury should always be suspected in a patient who has had a road traffic accident (RTA) and is in shock or after any kind of penetrating injury such as a knife or gunshot wound.

TYPES OF INJURY

When the artery is completely transected the diagnosis is usually straightforward. Lacerations, dissections, and contusions are usually missed or diagnosed late. Types of injuries may be:

- arterial,
- venous,
- associated fractures and nerve damage,
- arteriovenous fistulas,
- false aneurysms (Figure 2.3.1).

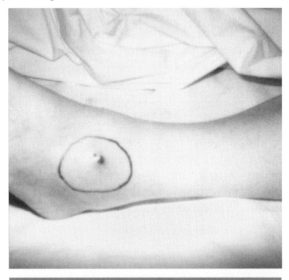

Fig. 2.3.1: A false aneurysm of the anterior tibial artery following injury during ankle arthroscopy.

PATHOPHYSIOLOGY

Patients with vascular trauma are usually young males with lower limb injuries involved in RTA, knife or gunshot wounds. The classic examples are communuted fracture of the femur, open tibial fracture with transection of artery and vein with extensive damage to muscle, soft tissues and contamination. Pathophysiological sequelae is as below:

Injured $\rightarrow$ Reduced $\rightarrow$ Reduced $\rightarrow$ Ischaemia–reperfusion
artery   perfusion   oxygen   injury

$\rightarrow$ Increased $\rightarrow$ Arterial
    capillary   repair
    permeability

RESUSCITATION

It is essential that resuscitation should precede diagnosis in patients with multiple serious injuries. These patients are usually bleeding, pale, apprehensive and short of breath.

- Follow general advanced trauma life support (ATLS) guidelines.
- Control of external bleeding with finger, pressure dressing, or pressure artery proximal to the bleeding point.
- Never attempt to blindly clamp the artery deep in the wound.
- For chest injuries, consider chest drain before assisted ventilation.
- For serious thoracic injuries cardiothoracic surgeon should be involved early.
- For abdominal injuries, general surgical team need to be contacted.

SITES OF INJURY

Chest and abdomen

More than 15% of deaths after motor vehicle accidents are caused by rupture of the thoracic aorta. Blunt injury may also fracture ribs and cause bleeding from the intercostal arteries into the pleural cavity. Penetrating thoracic trauma may damage the superior and inferior vena cava, the pulmonary artery and vein, and the aorta or its major branches.

Limb injury

Different signs and symptoms may be associated with extremity vascular injury depending on the site, mechanism, and extent of injury. Blunt limb trauma usually involves head and torso, and upper limb trauma causes extensive nerve damage.

DIAGNOSIS

Early angiography is necessary in blunt and complex penetrating trauma, as the clinical examination is unreliable. Ideal management of penetrating extremity trauma with the presence of at least one hard sign is immediate transfer to the operating theatre after initial resuscitation (Figure 2.3.2).

SIGNS OF VASCULAR INJURY

Hard signs

- Absent pulses.
- Bruit or thrill.
- Active haemorrhage.
- Haematoma (large).
- Distal ischaemia.

Soft signs

- Haematoma (small).
- History of haemorrhage at scene.
- Unexplained hypotension.
- Peripheral nerve deficit.

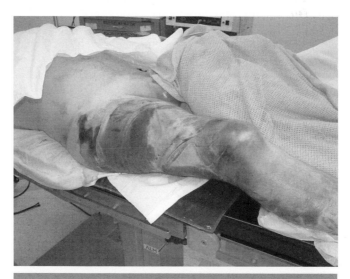

Fig. 2.3.2: A crush injury of the right leg that required amputation.

Soft signs are not particularly useful in the diagnosis of vascular injury. The role of non-invasive duplex scan or angiography is useful in these patients.

OPERATIVE MANAGEMENT

Majority of the patients will require surgical exploration and repair.

- The principles of emergency vascular repair are to control life-threatening haemorrhage and prevent limb ischaemia.
- More than 6–8 h of warm ischaemia time makes limb survival, despite revascularisation unlikely.
- In general, severe head injury and life-threatening haemorrhage from chest or abdomen takes precedence over limb trauma.
- The decision to perform primary amputation is difficult and complex and should be multi-disciplinary.
- Fasciotomy should be considered early, with limb trauma particularly when involving bones and muscles injuries.

REFERENCES

Barros D'Sa AAB (1998) How do we manage acute limb ischaemia due to trauma? In: Greenhalgh RM, Jamieson CW, Nocolaides AN (eds). *Limb Salvage and Amputation for Vascular Disease*. WB Saunders, London; p. 135.

Blaisdell FW, Steele M & Allen RE (1978). Management of lower extremity arterial ischaemic due to embolism and thrombosis. *Surgery* 84: 822–834.

Johnston KW (1994). Ruptured abdominal aortic aneurysm: six year follow up results of a multicentre prospective study – Canadian Society for Vascular Surgery Aneurysm Study Group. *J Vasc Surg* 19: 888–900.

Regel G, Lobenhoffer P, Grotz M, Pape HC, Lehmann U & Tscheme H (1995) Treatment results of patients with multiple trauma: an analysis of 3406 cases treated between 1972 and 1991 at a German Level I Trauma Centre. *J Trauma* 38(1): 70–8.

Sayers RD, Thompson MM, Varty K, Jagger C & Bell PRF (1993). Changing trends in the management of lower-limb ischaemia: a 17-year review. *Br J Surg* 80(10): 1269–1273.

3

VASCULAR INVESTIGATIONS

3.1 THE VASCULAR LABORATORY

C. Spencer

WHAT IS A VASCULAR LABORATORY?

A vascular laboratory is a hospital department in which non-invasive vascular assessments (NIVA) are carried out. These are mainly advanced ultrasound techniques using colour duplex and Doppler ultrasound. Other tests include plethysmography and segmental pressure measurements. In recent years the equipment has become more advanced making the investigations more accurate, safer and more cost effective (see Figure 3.1.1).

Ultrasound (conventional)

This provides anatomical information of the vessel being examined. An example of use is the monitoring and measurement of aortic aneurysms.

High frequency sound waves created by passing a current through a piezo-electric element are transmitted via a transducer into tissue and the reflected sound is used to form an image, based on a time base, which can be displayed on a monitor (Figure 3.1.2).

Doppler ultrasound

This is used to measure the direction and velocity of flow within a vessel. It can also be used to measure the volume of flow within a vessel.

Doppler ultrasound takes its name from the Austrian physicist Christian Doppler (1803–1853) who was the first person to identify the effect on sound as the wavelength changes, i.e. Doppler effect. The Doppler effect can be heard frequently in our daily lives. An example being the apparent change in pitch of an emergency vehicle as it approaches. This is because as the vehicle moves towards you the frequency of the sound waves reaching you is increased resulting in a change in tone of the signal.

As an ultrasound transducer is designed to both transmit and receive sound waves the Doppler effect occurs twice, once with the transmitted pulse to the tissue and other with the received pulse from the tissue. In vascular ultrasound the fact that the Doppler effect occurs twice enables us to monitor blood flow. The changes between the two pulses, i.e. the Doppler shift frequency detects the changes in the blood flow within the vessel.

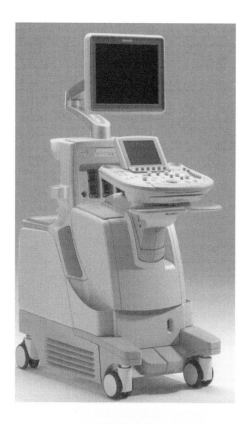

Fig. 3.1.1: The Philips iU22 ultrasound system.

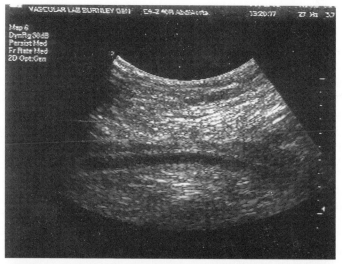

Fig. 3.1.2: Ultrasound scan of cross over femoro-femoral graft.

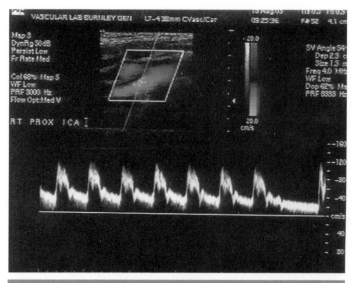

Fig. 3.1.3: A Duplex scan of the carotid artery bifurcation.

Duplex scan

This combines both conventional and Doppler ultrasound and therefore has the advantage of providing both dynamic and anatomical information (Figure 3.1.3).

Colour flow ultrasound

Colour is used to demonstrate the direction of the flow within the vessels. The colours used are usually red and blue with one colour showing flow towards the transducer and the other showing flow away from the transducer. Colour flow ultrasound is angle dependant where as power flow uses only one colour and shows flow regardless of direction. This is useful when there is only poor flow within a vessel. Colour is routinely used in Duplex scan machines (colour Duplex) (Figure 3.1.4).

Examinations

As ultrasound is a non-invasive procedure there is virtually no preparation needed prior to the scan except for an explanation to the patient of how the examination will be performed.

The exception to this includes: if the patient is excessively hirsute the area to be examined may require shaving (very rare). This is because in order for the

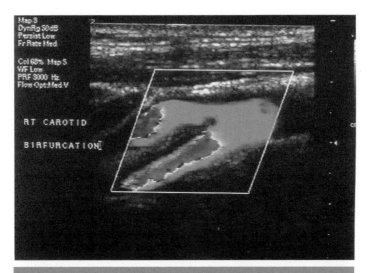

Fig. 3.1.4: Colour Duplex of the carotid bifurcation.

examination to be successful there needs to be a good contact between the skin and the surface of the transducer.

In order to improve this contact and eliminate an air gap between the skin and transducer a contact gel is applied to the area requiring investigation. (This is because air is a poor conductor of sound.)

In the case of investigations of the portal system the patient is required to starve completely for a period of 6 h prior to the scan. This prevents bowel gas and peristalsis obscuring the features to be scanned.

The aim of any vascular ultrasound examination is to determine the presence of any significant vascular disease. In arteries this is usually stenosis or occlusion of the vessels.

Arterial examination
In all investigations the vessels are examined with:

- *Ultrasound* to determine the size and condition of the vessels, and to detect the presence of any wall calcification or calcified plaque in arteries, or visible thrombus in veins.
- *Colour duplex* to show how well the vessels are filling and to outline any filling defect or plaque within the vessel. The type of plaque can also be determined

as either calcified, soft or ulcerative. The direction of flow within the vessel can also be ascertained.
- *Doppler* to determine the rate of flow in the vessel. Sample velocities are measured in several areas of the vessels and specifically in areas where there has been a stenosis identified with the colour duplex. The volume of flow through a stenosis can also be calculated.

The arteries examined are:

- Carotid arteries: Subclavian artery, common carotid artery, internal carotid artery, external carotid artery and the vertebral artery. Both sides are examined so that contra-lateral disease can be excluded.
- Lower limb arteries: Common iliac artery, external iliac artery, common femoral artery, superficial artery, popliteal artery and the tibial artery run-off at the trifurcation. Also examined are the origin of the internal iliac artery and the first few centimetres of the profunda artery. In the case of severe arterial disease, collateral flow is also identified.
- Upper limb arteries: Inominate artery, subclavian artery, axillary artery, brachial artery, radial and ulnar arteries.
- Abdominal arteries
  - The abdominal aorta for diagnosis and surveillance of aneurysms (Figures 3.1.5 and 3.1.6).
  - The renal arteries in investigations of renal artery stenosis. However, computed tomography (CT) or magnetic resonance arteriography (MRA) gives more accurate results.

Surveillance scans are also used:

- to assess the expansion of small aortic aneurysms at regular intervals (usually every 6 or 12 months);
- to detect stenosis in femoro-popliteal vein grafts.

Venous examination
Veins are examined for the presence of deep venous thrombus (DVT) and also for venous incompetence. Unlike arteries which have smooth inner wall, veins have valves to prevent the back flow of blood. Artery walls are rigid but vein walls are elastic in nature and can stretch to accommodate increased blood flow through the system. This property of veins can mean that they become over-stretched and the valve leaflets fail to close correctly allowing blood to flow back in the wrong direction, causing the so-called venous incompetence.

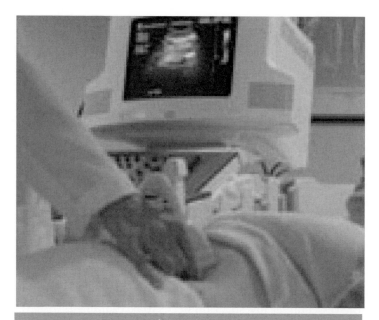

Fig. 3.1.5: Scanning of the abdominal aorta.

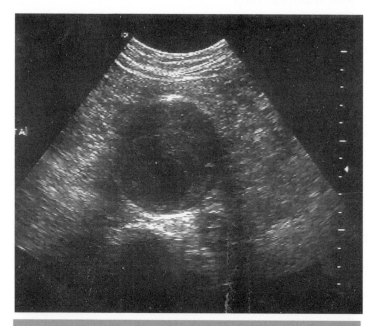

Fig. 3.1.6: US scan of an abdominal aortic aneurysm.

The vessels examined are:

- Lower limb: External iliac vein, common femoral vein, superficial femoral vein, popliteal vein, tibial veins, long and short saphenous veins. The sapheno-femoral and sapheno-popliteal junctions are also examined.
- Upper limb: Subclavian vein, axillary vein, brachial vein, radial and ulnar veins. In the examinations prior to or after access fistula formation the cephalic and basilic veins are investigated.

Advantages and disadvantages of colour Doppler ultrasound

Advantages
- It is a non-invasive procedure.
- It is cheaper and less labour intensive than conventional angiography.
- It does not require hospitalisation.
- It is quicker and less traumatic for the patient.
- Only the vessel under investigation needs to be examined.
- Only in rare cases is any preparation required.
- It is a good diagnostic tool eliminating the need for unnecessary procedures.
- There is no risk of radiation.

Disadvantages
- The procedures are only as good as the operator (it is important that the operator is fully trained in vascular ultrasound techniques and is fully conversant with the equipment).
- Examinations may be unreliable because of factors affecting the quality of the scan, e.g. if the patient is unable to keep still.
- Vessel wall calcification can lead to misdiagnosis of occlusions (calcification affects the reflectivity of the sound wave).
- Physical difficulties can prevent accurate measurements being made.

KEY POINTS

The roles of the vascular laboratory are as follows:

- Diagnosis and assessment of vascular disease.
- Pre- and postoperative monitoring and surveillance.
- Helps the doctor to select the required treatment.

FURTHER READING

MEDLINEplus Medical Encyclopaedia. Found at www.nlm.nih.gov/medlineplus

Oates C. *Cardiovascular Haemodynamics*. Greenwhich Medical Media, Cambridge University Press.

Thrush A, Hartshorne T. *Peripheral Vascular Ultrasound, How, Why and When*. Churchill Livingstone, 1999.

Other useful websites
www.worldwidewounds.com
www.crc.ed.ac.uk

3.2 RADIOLOGICAL INVESTIGATION AND INTERVENTION

W. Stevenson

INTRODUCTION

Diagnostic and interventional vascular radiology is one of the most rapidly growing fields in medicine today.

The development of the modern balloon catheter for angioplasty by Gruntzig in the 1970s was an important step in converting vascular radiology from a predominantly diagnostic into a therapeutic one.

More recent innovations in imaging and angiographic equipments as well as catheters, stents and stent grafts have led to the fact that minimally invasive techniques are being used more frequently to treat patients with peripheral vascular disease.

MINIMALLY INVASIVE INVESTIGATION

Most patients are still managed in a district general hospital (DGH) setting by clinical and radiology department staff who have other responsibilities than "vascular" patients. It is intended that care will evolve towards fewer number of larger specialist units, comparable to those in place in the larger centres. The transition may take many years. The diagnostic and treatment pathway for a patient depends on local practices and resources.

Although ultrasound (US) is less labour intensive than angiography it should not be employed indiscriminately, but it is harmless, and in combination with history and examination will usually demonstrate presence and absence of significant disease separately in the aortoiliac, femoropopliteal and distal segments. Angiography is rarely required for further diagnosis. US is usually carried out by radiographers from the X-ray department, but may be under the auspices of a vascular laboratory.

Computed tomography (CT) angiography is frequently requested for preoperative assessment of aortic aneurysm, and follow-up of radiological endovascular aneurysm repair. When proximal major vessels are occluded and conventional angiography is not feasible, CT can demonstrate the distal vessels beyond the blockage to aid surgical planning for bypass (Figure 3.2.1). It requires

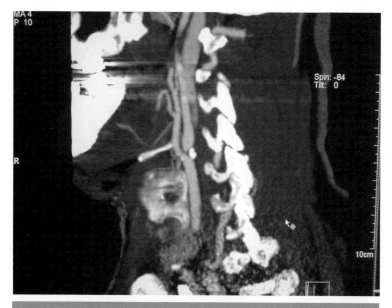

Fig. 3.2.1: CT angiogram of the carotid artery demonstrating a tight stenosis at the origin of the internal carotid artery with a calcified plaque.

intravenous contrast pumped through a cannula in a peripheral vein and the usual caution is necessary regarding interaction with metformin in renal failure, and the exceedingly rare and unpredictable severe contrast reaction. Rarely, contrast is extravasated into the soft tissues but this is unlikely to lead to problems.

Magnetic resonance imaging (MRI) angiography can provide similar information to CT, but there are essentially no contrast risks. Some patients are unable to tolerate the feeling of confinement inside the magnet bore. Time on the machine is in great demand because of the numerous applications in many aspects of medical care, providing information which often cannot be obtained by other investigations.

CONVENTIONAL ANGIOGRAPHY

Patients arrive at this stage when it is felt that "something must be done" either for intractable limiting claudication or critical ischaemia with rest pain and/or the prospect of amputation. The aim is to avert surgery either for amputation or surgical bypass, or to aid planning for surgery.

In some centres many radiological interventional procedures are performed as day cases (Macdonald *et al.*, 2002), which requires a suitable infrastructure, but in other places much of the work involves in-patients with severe vascular disease, and other medical and social problems. In many critical cases the patients are very unfit, and it becomes worthwhile to expend a lot of time and effort in the hope of improving limb vascular supply even when there is a low probability of success, because it is unlikely that "things will be made worse".

Pre-assessment may take place in the out-patient department (OPD) to determine suitability for a day-case procedure, and consent may be obtained unless it is policy to obtain this immediately prior to the procedure. Blood tests may be taken, including investigation for clotting abnormalities.

It is important to note diabetes, metformin treatment (http://www.rcr.ac.uk/pubtop.asp?PublicationID = 70), renal function, severe uncorrected hypertension, antiplatelet (aspirin) and anticoagulant (warfarin) treatment, recent cardiac and cerebral vascular events. These may constitute relative or absolute contraindications to a procedure, depending upon the condition of the patient. Factors such as the availability of recovery/observation space and nursing staff within the radiology department will determine local practices.

Prior to the procedure some radiologists require shaving off the groins and further blood tests. Sedation or intravenous analgesia is rarely indicated since patient alertness may protect against vessel rupture during angioplasty. Access

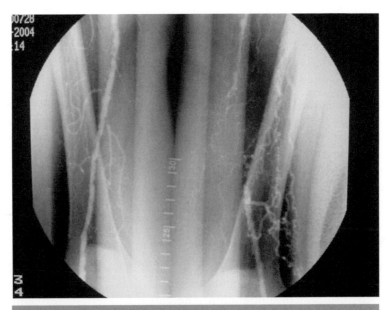

Fig. 3.2.2: Conventional angiography of the femoral arteries. Note the occlusion in the left superficial femoral artery.

to the arterial system is usually by puncture of femoral artery at the groin, brachial artery at the elbow or rarely the axillary artery, following infiltration with local anaesthetic. A wire is passed to the desired position, and a catheter passed along the wire. Contrast is injected and images recorded; if a stenosis or occlusion is identified, with reasonable vessels beyond "runoff" then angioplasty may be considered (Figure 3.2.2).

BALLOON ANGIOPLASTY

Balloon angioplasty was pioneered by Gruentzig (1984) for the coronary circulation and later applied to the peripheral circulation. Technical advances have produced superb balloons of numerous diameters which can tolerate inflation pressures around 15 atm and which require only a small entry hole in the artery. Balloon inflation painfully ruptures the stenosing plaque, generally without rupturing the outer wall of the vessel. Even complete rupture is recoverable (Hayes *et al.*, 2002), either by radiological methods or the aid of the vascular surgeon.

The original technique involved finding the true vessel lumen and dilating it up, but Bolia and Leicester vascular group invented and promulgated the sub-intimal route (London *et al.*, 1994), which had previously been considered an undesirable "dissection". A slippery coated wire is deliberately introduced into the original wall of the vessel which surrounds what may be a completely occluded lumen; for instance, the entire length of the superficial femoral artery may be blocked and therefore invisible on the angiogram, and yet a long lasting functional channel may be created by this method. The procedure is technically difficult and some operators have more success than others.

Occlusion and stenosis may well recur, but this is less likely in the larger vessels, such as the iliac arteries. This may be dilated again or a stent may be placed (Figure 3.2.3).

Complications

- *Technical failure*: patient no worse off, apart from the pain and discomfort of the procedure.
- *Vessel rupture*: possibly with concealed retroperitoneal bleeding and may be requiring surgery.
- *Worsening of ischaemia*: leading to emergency surgery.
- *Continued bleeding* at the groin with formation of visible haematoma: firm digital pressure.
- *Myocardial infarction (MI), stroke and death*: these patients usually have extensive cardiovascular disease, and are at risk for these events even without the stress of a long vascular procedure.

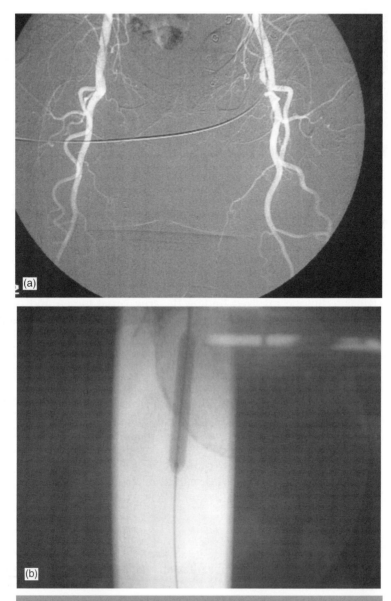

Fig. 3.2.3: Balloon angioplasty of the right superficial femoral artery.

Aftercare

- Observe and question the patient. Do not cover the puncture sites.
- Monitor blood pressure (BP) and pulse rate at agreed intervals.

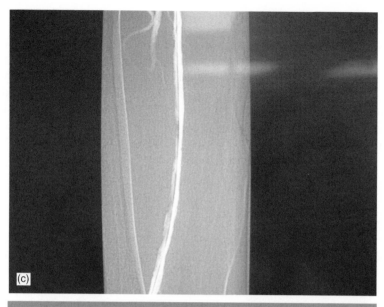

Fig. 3.2.3: (Continued)

- Day case: bed rest for 1 or 2 h, out of bed and home after agreed process of assessment.
- In-patient: often not ambulant in any case. Review by vascular specialist team or radiology staff.

CAROTID ARTERY ANGIOPLASTY AND STENTING

Carotid artery disease may result in specific types of cerebral ischaemic events (see Chapter 1). Indications for carotid endarterectomy are evolving (Rothwell and Warlow, 1999; Naylor *et al.*, 2003), based on various factors including information on degree of stenosis provided by US or CT carotid angiography. Alternative treatments include antiplatelet drugs, and carotid angioplasty and stenting (Gaines, 2000) which is carried out in major centres as part of controlled trials, even as a day case (Tan *et al.*, 2003). Angioplasty may cause cerebral embolic events like those occurring during heart bypass for coronary artery grafting. The risk may be reduced by neuroprotective devices which trap small particles before they reach the brain (Macdonald and Gaines, 2003), but the procedure competes with endarterectomy carried out under local anaesthetic with an awake patient who can alert the surgeon to problems, and who may well be discharged home the following day.

ENDOVASCULAR ANEURYSM REPAIR

Endovascular repair of abdominal aortic aneurysm (EVAR) (Thomas *et al.*, 2001) is a difficult procedure also restricted to specialist units and controlled trials to allow accumulation of expertise. Indications change with technical advance in the devices, but include patients unfit or unwilling to undergo operative repair. Large units may offer the procedure on an emergency basis. Extensive CT follow-up is required to monitor blood leaks into the aneurysm sac and other complications.

GLOSSARY

Conventional angiography – Takes place on a table which moves in relation to an X-ray tube which can be angled to display vascular lesions in profile. It may take several hours if interventional procedures are performed, and after care may well be required. Involves all the cumbersome paraphernalia of a "sterile" procedure and usually involves an admission, even if only as a "day case". Contrast is injected into an artery by a pump at about 10 ml/s. Quick and easy digital "subtraction" removes the dense bone from the image, leaving clear pictures of the vessels. It is very difficult or impossible with distal aortic or bilateral iliac artery occlusion. The radiation dose is kept to a minimum, but may be very high which is largely irrelevant for such patients. Angiography began in the 1930s but became widespread only in the 1960s.

CT scanning – A powerful X-ray tube rotates continuously around the long axis of the patient who moves slowly through the beam. Later machines acquire several (up to 16 at present) "slices" of the patient simultaneously, and this rapid imaging allows *CT* angiography with intravenous contrast at a rate of up to 5 ml/s. Very high radiation dose is not significant for those patients who actually need the examination. The scans are quick to perform but easily comprehensible display of the vessels requires time-consuming computer manipulation of the many hundreds of slices, to remove interfering bone without introducing significant error. No after care is required. It can show distal "run-off" vessels even with proximal arterial occlusion. Clinical computed tomography scanners were introduced in late 1970s (Figures 3.2.4 and 3.2.5).

MRI – The latest of the "scanners" employs a combination of extremely strong magnetic fields, radiowave energy (non-ionising electromagnetic radiation) and massive computing power to image all parts of the body with innumerable techniques to emphasise differing tissues and pathologies. Clinical scanners are completely harmless, but scans are time consuming, noisy and usually take place in the confined space inside a cylindrical magnet – some patients

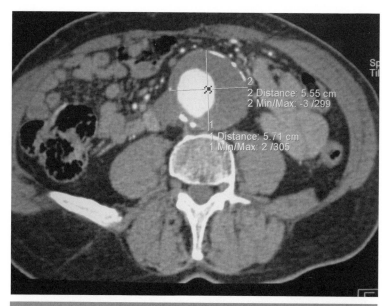

Fig. 3.2.4: CT scan of an abdominal aortic aneurysm.

are unable to tolerate this. There are numerous ways to demonstrate the vascular system, both with and without "contrast". No after care is required. It can show distal "run-off" vessels even with proximal arterial occlusion. *MRI has become increasingly important since clinical introduction in the 1980s* (Figure 3.2.6).

Contrast – A substance which is introduced into the body to display the desired anatomy; here, it is injected into, and shows the lumen of blood vessels. Arteriography, venography, computed tomography, conventional angiography and intravenous urography all employ contrast which (like bone) transmits X-rays less well than soft tissues; therefore contrast containing blood vessels stand out with a similar density to bone. Such contrast is now invariably of the "non-ionic" variety with much reduced symptoms of heat and nausea after injection – a very small risk of anaphylaxis remains, but most radiologists have never seen a serious contrast reaction.

It is suggested that there is a risk of severe reaction between these contrast agents and diabetic patients taking metformin (http://www.rcr.ac.uk/pubtop. asp?PublicationID = 70), resulting in kidney damage. In practice, problems only arise in patients with pre-existing renal impairment (Nawaz *et al.*, 1998), and the present practice is to discontinue metformin prior to contrast injection and only recommence 2 days later if renal function tests are "normal".

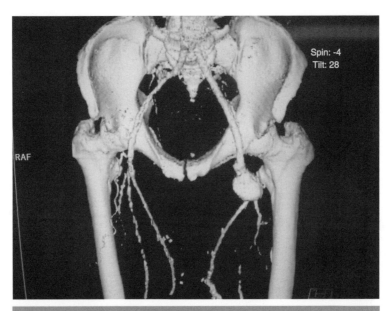

Spin: -4
Tilt: 28

RAF

Fig. 3.2.5: A spiral CT angiogram of an aorto-bifemoral graft and bilateral femoro-popliteal bypass grafts. This patient presented with a large pulsatile swelling in the left groin 15 years after he had had the above procedures and the CT angiogram confirmed the presence of a false aneurysm of the left common femoral artery.

Stent – Expandable metal framework visible on the television screen, mounted on a delivery device, such as a catheter, which allows passage along a guide wire to the desired position within the vessel. The aim is to maintain the newly created or expanded lumen. The frame may be covered in order to seal a hole in the vessel. Amazing technical advances, driven by the vast market for stenting of the coronary arteries, have produced stents which slowly release drugs to reduce in-stent restenosis (Gunn *et al.*, 2003). These are not yet employed in the larger peripheral arteries.

Ultrasound – Sound waves much higher in frequency than the 20 kHz threshold of human hearing – usually around 5 MHz. Black and white images are produced by reflection of sound waves at various soft tissue interfaces within the body, and ultrasound is unable to image around air and bone. The Doppler effect and other properties are employed to identify moving blood and portray it as colour on the image. It is completely harmless, and in medical use since the 1960s.

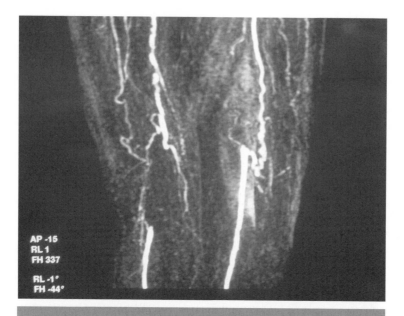

Fig. 3.2.6: MR angiogram of the superficial femoral arteries.

X-rays – They are part of the electromagnetic spectrum which includes radiowaves, microwaves, infrared, visible light and ultraviolet. X-rays are more energetic and potentially more harmful than any of these, and are described as ionising radiation from the ability to knock outermost electrons from the gas molecules in air to produce positively charged ions. This property corresponds to a potential to damage intracellular components, such as DNA, and therefore harm the patient. Discovered by Roentgen in 1895, and used within months to diagnose fractures.

Thrombolysis is the treatment to dissolve blood clots that are blocking blood vessels (arteries or veins). The procedure is carried out by introducing a lytic agent directly into the clot through a catheter. Two thrombolytic agents commonly used are urokinase and altepase (tissue plasminogen activator, t-PA).

Embolisation is the procedure where various substances are used (via a catheter) to reduce or completely occlude blood flow through an artery. It may be used as a primary treatment to control bleeding (e.g. gastrointestinal bleeding) or arterio-venous malformations or as an adjunctive treatment to chemotherapy or radiotherapy in the management of certain tumours. Materials used for embolisation include coils, ethanol, polyvinyl alcohol and gelatin sponge.

REFERENCES

Davies A, on behalf of the PVD working party (2000) The practical management of claudication. *Br Med J* 321: 911–912.

Gaines PA (2000) Carotid angioplasty and stenting. *Br Med Bull* 56(2): 549–556.

Gruentzig AR (1984) Percutaneous transluminal coronary angioplasty: six years' experience. *Am Heart J* 107(4): 818–819.

Guidelines with Regard to Metformin-Induced Lactic Acidosis and X-ray Contrast Medium Agents, http://www.rcr.ac.uk/pubtop.asp?PublicationID = 70

Gunn J, Grech ED, Crossman D & Cumberland D (2003) New developments in percutaneous coronary intervention. *Br Med J* 327: 150–153.

Hayes PD, Chokkalingam A, Jones R, Bell PR, Fishwick G, Bolia A & Naylor AR (2002) Arterial perforation during infrainguinal lower limb angioplasty does not worsen outcome: results from 1409 patients. *J Endovasc Ther* 9(4): 422–427.

London NJ, Srinivasan R, Naylor AR, Hartshorne T, Ratliff DA, Bell PR & Bolia A (1994) Subintimal angioplasty of femoropopliteal artery occlusions: the long-term results. *Eur J Vasc Surg* 8(2): 148–155.

Macdonald S & Gaines PA (2003) Current concepts of mechanical cerebral protection during percutaneous carotid intervention. *Vasc Med* 8(1): 25–32.

Macdonald S, Thomas SM, Cleveland TJ & Gaines PA (2002) Outpatient vascular intervention: a two-year experience. *Cardiovasc Intervent Radiol* 25(5): 403–412.

Nawaz S, Cleveland T, Gaines PA & Chan P (1998) Clinical risk associated with contrast angiography in metformin treated patients: a clinical review. *Clin Radiol* 53(5): 342–344.

Naylor AR, Rothwell PM & Bell PR (2003) Overview of the principal results and secondary analyses from the European and North American randomised trials of endarterectomy for symptomatic carotid stenosis. *Eur J Vasc Endovasc Surg* 26(2): 115–129.

Rothwell PM & Warlow CP, on behalf of the European Carotid Surgery Trialists' Collaborative Group (1999) Prediction of benefit from carotid endarterectomy in individual patients: a risk-modelling study. *Lancet* 353: 2105–2110.

Tan KT, Cleveland TJ, Berczi V, McKevitt FM, Venables GS & Gaines PA (2003) Timing and frequency of complications after carotid artery stenting: what is the optimal period of observation? *J Vasc Surg* 38(2): 236–243.

Thomas SM, Gaines PA & Beard JD, Vascular Surgical Society of Great Britain and Ireland, and British Society of Interventional Radiology (2001) Short-term (30-day) outcome of endovascular treatment of abdominal aortic aneurysm: results from the prospective Registry of Endovascular Treatment of Abdominal Aortic Aneurysm (RETA). *Eur J Vasc Endovasc Surg* 21(1): 57–64.

MANAGEMENT OF VASCULAR
PATIENTS ON THE WARD

4.1 NURSING CARE OF PATIENTS WITH PERIPHERAL VASCULAR DISEASE

S. Jane and S. Dorgan

INTRODUCTION

Caring for the patient with peripheral vascular disease (PVD) poses a challenge for nurses, as these patients do not always present with PVD in isolation. Many patients also suffer from diabetes and cardiac conditions. Partial or complete occlusion of a vessel results in reduced blood flow, causing oedema and congestion within the tissues (Watson & Royal, 1987). Pain experienced by vascular patients can be unrelenting and difficult to control.

Patients presenting with PVD need a thorough assessment of their needs and subsequent care provided by nurses with an understanding of vascular disease. This chapter addresses some of the problems encountered by patients with PVD and outlines the nursing care required for certain procedures and operations.

ACUTE AND CRITICAL LIMB ISCHAEMIA

- A sudden onset of severe pain as a result of an occlusion of an artery or vein will result in the patient requiring immediate treatment.
- On admission the patient should be urgently assessed by medical staff.
- Patients may be admitted from a variety of settings, to include the outpatients clinic, by general practitioner (GP) referral, accident and emergency department, from home or a specialist unit, such as renal or diabetes clinics.

Nursing care
The aim of nursing care is to establish a baseline for further recordings.

Rationale
The rationale includes the following:

- Assessment of the affected limb, including skin colour, temperature, presence or absence of pulses, and pain.

- There may be a notable difference in colour depending on the volume of blood being able to flow through the vessel. This should be accurately recorded (i.e. red, blue, dusky, blotchy and how far it extends).
- Capillary refill can be checked by blanching the skin for 5 s and then releasing. The veins should refill in approximately 3–5 s.
- In the lower limb, pulses should be located, palpated and recorded as present or absent.

Following the assessment, the patient may require urgent surgical attention. However, surgery may not be necessary if an urgent angiogram is performed with a resulting angioplasty which may rectify the problem. This can be performed in the radiology department or in the operating theatre.

ELECTIVE ANGIOGRAPHY

An angiogram is an X-ray procedure enabling diagnosis of a blockage or malfunction in the arteries. It provides the vascular team with knowledge of the extent and location of any arterial disease. A needle and small catheter is inserted into the artery at the groin. Contrast (dye) is injected down the catheter and X-rays taken as the solution passes along the arteries. These X-rays can be used to determine patients' treatment plans.

Pre-procedure
- The patient is often admitted on the day of the procedure.
- Individual hospital guidelines should be adhered to in terms of:
  - fasting,
  - stopping anticoagulant therapy,
  - monitoring of diabetes,
  - preparation of the groin region prior to procedure.
- Informed consent needs to be given by the patient once the negative and positive aspects of the procedure have been explained.
- Any special instructions should be relayed to the radiology staff; e.g. problems with the patients mobility, such as arthritis, spinal conditions or chronic obstructive airways disease; all of which may affect whether the patient can lie flat.

Post-procedure
- The patient is returned to the ward where observation is continued for several hours.
- Individual hospital guidelines should be adhered to in terms of:
  - the number of hours for which the patient should lie flat;
  - the recording of blood pressure (BP) and pulse;
  - observation of the puncture site.

ANGIOPLASTY

This is a procedure in which a balloon is passed into the artery on the end of a catheter, then inflated to treat a narrowed or blocked artery. The inflated balloon breaks the plaque, pushes it back against the artery wall, stretches the artery and subsequently increases the blood flow. The catheter is then removed once the balloon has been deflated. If the artery has been sufficiently stretched (determined by injecting contrast dye), it means that the need for surgery is avoided (albeit temporarily in some cases). Nursing care is similar to that following angiography.

CAROTID ENDARTERECTOMY

A narrowing or occlusion of the carotid arteries is a potentially life-threatening condition which if not monitored or rectified by surgery can be fatal.

One of the major concerns for patients undergoing this type of surgery is the possible complication of stroke.

Carotid endarterectomy is now commonly performed to help prevent stroke in high-risk patients.

Pre-operative investigations
- Blood screening.
- A carotid duplex scan is often performed to ascertain the extent and percentage of the stenosis in the arteries. Both sides of the carotid may be affected but the patient usually has only one side operated on at a time.
- Chest X-ray
- Angiogram may be requested depending on the local policy.
- Electrocardiogram (ECG).

Rationale
These investigations will offer insight at the patients' level of fitness and suitability to undergo surgery.

Pre-operative health education
- Stopping smoking.
- Reducing BP.
- Weight loss.
- Reduction of alcohol intake.
- Reduction of cholesterol.
- Control of diabetes.

Rationale

By addressing the listed issues, the patient should aim to be as fit as possible prior to the surgical procedure.

Pre-operative care

According to the local guidelines the pre-operative care includes the following:

1. Nursing and medical assessments.
2. Sliding scale of insulin if patient has diabetes.
3. Baseline observations of BP, pulse, temperature, blood tests, chest X-ray and ECG.
4. Offering of pre-medication if required to reduce anxiety.
5. Informed consent.
6. Cross-match or group and save.
7. Nil by mouth prior to surgery.
8. Give oral medication even if nil by mouth, especially antihypertensive drugs.
9. Visit to high-dependency area if appropriate.

The surgery can be performed under local or general anaesthesia. Details of the surgery are found in Chapter 5.

Post-operative complications

Post-operative complications can include:

1. Hypertension.
2. Hypotension.
3. Haemorrhage.
4. Cranial nerve injury.
5. Cerebrovascular accident (CVA).

Hypertension

Blood Pressure fluctuation can occur as a result of interruption or injury to the carotid sinus nerve. Hypertension increases the risk of other post-operative complications like haematoma and hyperperfusion syndrome. For example, careful assessment should determine the cause of the rise in BP, as it may be a physiological response to pain. Alert the medical team if all other possible causes have been ruled out, as antihypertensives and vasodilators may be required.

Hypotension

A fall in BP, accompanied by tachycardia may indicate haemorrhage, which requires immediate action. Hypotension can predispose the patient to coronary artery thrombosis and any existing cardiac disease may be complicated by extremes in BP.

Haemorrhage

This is usually the result of overdose of anticoagulants, leakage from the arterial line suture and inadequate surgical techniques (Ginzberg *et al.*, 1997). However, major bleeding after this operation is uncommon – <1% of patients. A blood-soaked dressing is the first manifestation of wound bleeding. Nurses should observe for bleeding, record and report if observed, ensure the dressing is clean and secure, and check if the drain is patent and draining. A coagulation profile should be initiated to rule out overdose of anticoagulants.

Nerve injury

Nerve injuries may result from traction, inadvertent clamping or unskilled use of electrocautery. Observation is often the best intervention, as 80% of nerve impairments resolve within 3 months, although 7% are permanent (Gough *et al.*, 1999). Sixteen per cent of patients may suffer cranial nerve damage. Therefore, nurses should assess for any damage by noting any voice changes (indicating recurrent laryngeal nerve damage), deviation of the tongue towards the side of the operation (hypoglossal injuries) and drooping of the lip ipsilateral to the surgery (marginal mandibular injuries) (Hertzer, 1989).

Cerebrovascular accident

Embolic debris from the surgery site or new thrombus may become dislodged and lead to stroke.

ABDOMINAL AORTIC ANEURYSM

Aneurysms are irreversible dilatations of the arterial wall involving all layers.

- The vessel wall affected gradually increases in size and may rupture.
- Aneurysms are often detected during routine examinations for surgery in other areas or routine ultrasound scans.
- Patients are often asymptomatic for years until the aneurysm increases in size.
- There are various forms of aneurysm.
- Patients found to have an aneurysm will be monitored by screening and once the patient becomes symptomatic or the size reaches 5.5 cm, surgery will be considered.

Elective surgical repair

The following investigations are usually performed:

- Myocardial infarction is the major cause of death after this form of surgery. Therefore, it is essential to assess cardiac and pulmonary status pre-operatively. This can significantly reduce the morbidity and mortality of the elective procedure.

- Blood count, urea and electrolytes, group and save serum, glucose, liver function tests and coagulation screen.
- Chest X-ray, ECG and echocardiogram.
- Routine scans should have already identified the size of the aneurysm.

Pre-operative care

- Routine medical and nursing assessments.
- Review by anaethetist.
- Baseline observations.
- Doppler assessment.
- Blood glucose monitoring if patient is diabetic.
- Pressure risk assessment.
- Consent for surgery.
- Written patient information leaflet detailing surgery and post-operative care.
- Nil by mouth prior to surgery.
- Offer visit to intensive care/high-dependency unit.

Post-operative care

The patient will be transferred to a critical care or high-dependency bed. Monitoring of vital signs, heart, lung and respiratory function will help detect any complications (see Chapter 2). Patients are observed for:

- Fluid balance: Patients are often kept nil by mouth for the first 24 h. Sips of water are then introduced building up to diet and fluids according to local policies. Patients undergoing this form of surgery are at high risk of developing a paralytic ileus, due to handling of the bowel during surgery. If the patient develops abdominal distension, pain and discomfort, the nil by mouth status may have to be reinstated.
- Respiratory status: Patients should be nursed in a semi-recumbent position and then upright as soon as possible to deter respiratory complications. Patients who smoke are at high risk of developing chest infections. A large, abdominal incision will add to this risk.
- Cardiovascular status.
- Renal status.
- Potential haemorrhage.
- Shock.
- Limb observations: Limb perfusion should be monitored and recorded, which involves palpating the dorsalis pedis and posterior tibial using

a hand-held Doppler. The nurse receiving the patient from theatre should establish the limb perfusion on leaving the theatre.

- Mobility: The patient should be mobilised as soon as possible following surgery to prevent complications of deep vein thrombosis, pulmonary embolism and the prevention of pressure ulcers.
- Wound care: The wound will usually be closed with staples on a transverse incision. The dressing and surrounding skin should be observed for signs of infection.
- The patient is often discharged home within 7–10 d. Advice on the need for rest, healthy diet and lifestyle should be reinforced on discharge.

ARTERIAL RECONSTRUCTIVE SURGERY OF THE LOWER LIMB

Some examples of possible sites for reconstructive surgery are given in Chapter 5.3. Revascularisation involves using a synthetic graft or an autogenous vein graft. Indications for bypass surgery vary and more details can be found in Chapter 5.3 (surgical procedures).

Pre-operative investigations
Pre-operative investigations may include:

- Duplex ultrasonography.
- Arteriography/computerised tomography (CT) angiogram.
- Blood tests.
- Chest X-ray.
- ECG.
- Baseline observations of BP, pulse, temperature, blood glucose (if diabetic) and respiratory function tests (if co-existing pulmonary disease).

Pre-operative nursing care
Pre-operative nursing care may include:

- Understanding of forthcoming procedure.
- Informed consent.
- Pain assessment.
- Nutritional needs.
- Pressure relief assessment.
- Nil by mouth as per local protocol.
- Assessment of needs on discharge (e.g. social services).

Post-operative nursing care

Post-operative nursing care may include:

- Continual haemodynamic monitoring.
- Limb observations (colour, temperature and presence of pedal pulses).
- Diet and fluid intake.
- Observation for any infection.
- Observation for haematoma and haemorrhage.
- Pain management;
- Pressure area relief.
- Preparation for safe discharge.

REFERENCES

Bick C, Imray C (2001) Carotid endarterectomy. *Nursing Stand* 16(3): 47–55.

Bick C, Imray C (2000) Abdominal aortic aneurysm repair. *Nursing Stand* 15(3): 47–52.

Timsit *et al.* (1992) Early clinical differentiation of cerebral infarction from severe artherosclerotic stenosis and cardio embolism. *Stroke* 23(4): 486–491.

Watson J, Royle JA (1987) *Medical–Surgical Nursing and related Physiology*. Baillière Tindall, London.

4.2 REHABILITATION OF AMPUTEES AND ARTIFICIAL LIMB PROVISION

F.J. Boon

INTRODUCTION

Amputation is performed to oblate disease and to provide an organ of function – usually for locomotion, as the majority of amputations for vascular disease are performed on the lower limb.

The latest UK statistics show that the majority of amputations are performed for disvascularity – arteriosclerosis followed by diabetes mellitus. The majority of these are performed at trans-tibial level followed by trans-femoral. There are nearly 6000 referrals to prosthetic services. Hospital activity analyses record 17,000 amputations are performed annually – a high proportion of these are digital amputations requiring little prosthetic intervention.

The majority of these patients are over 65-year-old with nearly a quarter over 75-year-old. Many have other complications associated with disvascularity – e.g. contra-lateral limb intermittent claudication, diabetic foot ulceration and charcot (neuropathic) joints – joints damaged as there is absent proprioception due to neuropathy.

Other organs are commonly involved and in this group patients often have a history of coronary heart disease (angina and heart failure), cerebrovascular accident (CVA), transient ischaemic attack (TIA), renal failure and diabetic retinopathy. Cognitive difficulties and dementia are common making it difficult for patients to understand and follow instructions with associated poor carry over from treatment sessions. In diabetes blood sugar control may be a problem, especially when the patient's activity may vary and hypoglycaemic episodes are not unusual. Resuscitation with glucose or occasionally dextrose or glucagon may be required to be injected.

It is worth remembering that a third of this patient group become double amputees before death.

REHABILITATION

Rehabilitation can be considered to begin immediately following surgery. Close attention at this stage can aid recovery and help with prosthetic rehabilitation.

Stump and phantom pain should be controlled. Patient-controlled analgesia (PCA) is commonly used initially, analgesia is later provided using the usual analgesic ladder and guidelines. Phantom sensation and pain initially affects most patients but often subsides in time. This requires to be explained to patients that it is not unusual or imaginary.

Each amputee suffers from an individual grief reaction to their loss, and sympathetic nursing team management is necessary.

Chest care should be undertaken and an exercise programme should be started.

Attention should be paid to pressure areas – sheep skins, cradles, special mattresses may be supplied.

Drains may be *in situ* and need to be managed. The type of stump dressing and compression regime vary – commonly a wool and crepe bandage dressing is used initially – later followed by a compression sock. These require close monitoring to avoid undue pressure thus avoiding tissue necrosis and delayed healing. Poor bandaging technique especially with a tight proximal constriction ring can produce or aggravate distal oedema.

MOBILISATION

Initially bed mobilisation is encouraged, perhaps with instruction on how to roll or pull up using a pulley or rope ladder tied to the bed end. Later transfers are practised – with assistance to begin with then self-transferring, sometimes managed with a sliding or banana board.

Wheelchair mobility needs to be taught – manoeuvre safely, apply brakes correctly and use a seatbelt. Pressure relieving cushions may be prescribed, such as a gel cushion. Double amputees need their rear wheels set back for greater stability. Patients not considered suitable for prostheses may be supplied with an electrically powered wheelchair.

Occupational therapists are required to give additional advice on activities of daily living – dressing, hygiene and toilet needs, plus arrange home visits with the patient and relatives to assess local environments.

PROSTHETIC PHASE

Immediate
Immediate post-operative prostheses (IPOP) are not commonly used in the UK, as there is a danger of tissue necrosis and wound breakdown.

Temporary

Pneumatic prostheses (e.g. post-amputation mobility (PAM) aid) are commonly used at both trans-tibial and trans-femoral levels. They can be used on the wards and also help in assessment and maintain and increase morale. Following this patients thought suitable for continuing prosthetic rehabilitation are referred for assessment to their local Disablement Services Centre (DSC).

The amputee service arose following the Great War when there was a large influx of new amputees. After World War II the service was managed by the Department of Health and Social Security (DHSS) and was fully integrated into the National Health Services (NHS) in 1990 following recommendations in the McColl report. Most DSCs are located in acute hospital sites and there are approximately 45 in the UK. Prostheses and accessories (e.g. stump socks) are provided and maintained at no cost to the patient.

Not all amputees are referred – some may choose not to try and others may be considered too weak or confused. In others a poor prognosis may not allow sufficient time. Occasionally their environment may be unsuitable, e.g. living in a mobile home.

Local stump problems, e.g. delayed healing may prevent early referral. Many stumps are not fully healed, even after 3 months. Local stump revision, such as shortening, wedge excision or conversion to a higher level is not infrequent. Stump oedema and joint contractures may require attention.

Energy requirements when walking with a prosthesis are high which is often the reason why the patients are advised not to use a prosthesis or abandon due to fatigue. A single below-knee amputee may need approximately 50% extra energy and for a single above-knee 100% extra energy may be required. These figures need to be at least doubled for bi-lateral loss (Figure 4.2.1).

Prosthetic construction

Modern prostheses are now mainly manufactured from plastics, carbon fibre and light alloys, and are of endoskeletal construction, i.e. with an internal skeleton, such as a carbon fibre shin tube to which other components are attached:

- Ankle and prosthetic socket in below-knee amputations (Figure 4.2.4).
- Ankle and prosthetic knee in above-knee prostheses.

Older prostheses were often made with an external skeleton (like an insect) which is called *exoskeletal construction*, e.g. a metal leg constructed like a tin can.

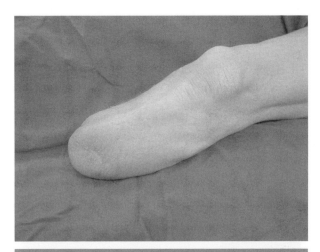

Fig. 4.2.1: A patient with a below knee amputation requires half the amount of energy compared to that of an above knee when walking with a prosthesis.

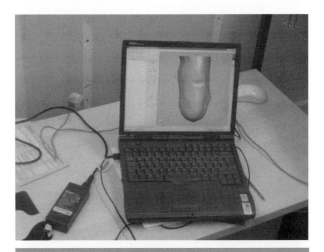

Fig. 4.2.2: Computer aided design has improved the quality of prosthetic limbs.

Lower limb prostheses are attached to the patient by means of a socket into which the stump is placed. Usually an interface is used, such as a cotton stump sock. The stump then controls the prosthesis. The socket transmits weight and may also help with suspension. Frequently additional suspension may be required, such as an elastic pelvic belt for above-knee amputees or a cuff strap for below-knee amputees (Figure 4.2.3). The socket design and shape is decided by the prosthetist and may be proximal weight bearing, such as the ischium taking weight in above-knee amputees or end bearing in Symes (through ankle amputation) or total surface bearing as in some below-knee sockets. Below-knee prostheses are often referred to as patella tendon bearing (PTB) as commonly some of the weight is taken over the patella tendon area.

The relationship between socket and shin tube, and ankle and foot can be altered by the prosthetist (alignment) to obtain maximum comfort function and cosmesis.

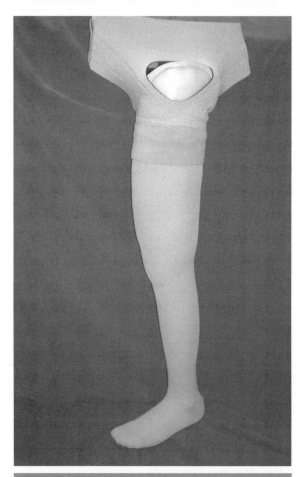

Fig. 4.2.3: An above knee prosthesis with a suspension belt.

Commonly patients wear a silicone sleeve as an interface with a prosthesis and for suspension a metal pin is attached to the sleeve which links into a shuttle lock which is an extremely secure form of suspension.

Prosthetic ankles and feet are of numerous design and they provide shock absorption with smooth roll over and sometimes assisted "toe off" with energy return.

Above-knee amputees require a knee unit – as the majority are elderly they are provided with a locked knee for ambulation which is unlocked by a button on the outer side of the socket. More active patients can be provided with an optional lock in addition to a free knee; e.g. if they are on rough terrain they can lock the knee. Very active patients are prescribed a free knee often with both stance and swing control. Stance control prevents the knee suddenly flexing – this is called "knee-shoot". Swing phase controls allow fine-tuning of the swing phase of the gait cycle and this is often provided by using pneumatic or hydraulic mechanisms. Some sophisticated knee units have microprocessor controls which adjust for varying walking speeds (cadence) automatically.

Additional components may be incorporated, such as torque absorbers which help to prevent shear forces with resultant skin trauma on the stump.

Long stumps may not allow sufficient room for all these components and occasionally external knee joints have to be provided for above-knee prostheses. These prostheses are of increased weight and have poor function and poor cosmesis. Other levels of amputation are less frequently encountered in vascular and diabetic patients, such as hip disarticulation, Symes and partial foot levels.

Double amputees

Below-knee patients are often initially provided with a pair of prostheses a fraction shorter than the patient's normal height to assist with balance.

Double above-knee amputees should be advised to become wheelchair mobile then occasionally they may attempt to use prostheses beginning with short rocker pylons before proceeding to a pair of definitive prostheses.

Patients who are unable to use a functional limb can opt for a foam cosmetic prosthesis and these can be very realistic.

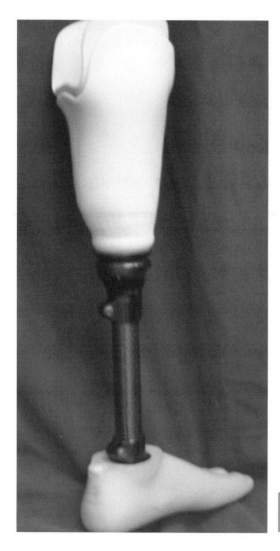

Fig. 4.2.4: A below knee modular prosthesis.

It is becoming more common to provide silicone cosmetic covers on prostheses and these are extremely realistic and life like.

Additional prostheses occasionally are required: e.g. waterproof prostheses for showering and water sports. Golfers often request a rotation unit to help with their swing!

For driving it is the patient's responsibility to contact the DVLA and sometimes special assessment at a driving centre is necessary. Commonly patients opt to drive with automatic transmission, as hand controls are quite difficult

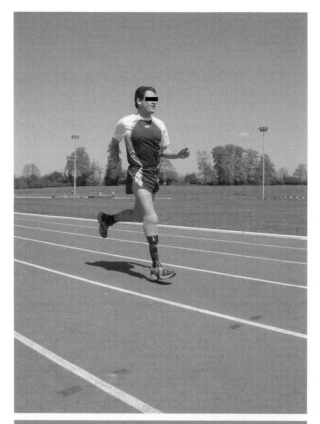

Fig. 4.2.5: Motivated young amputees can return to almost normal life style.

to manage. Once discharged home patients need the involvement of their general practitioner and community services to integrate and rehabilitate them (Figure 4.2.5).

Prostheses need regular maintenance and repair, and the majority of initial sockets require changing due to stump shrinkage.

Upper limb amputations

Upper limb amputations for disvascularity are relatively uncommon. Most are performed for trauma. Approximately 10% of arm amputees referred to DSC have had their amputation performed for disvascularity.

Rehabilitation depends on the patient's dominance and the level of loss. Some patients manage well without a prosthesis, others may try cosmetic or functional prostheses.

Functional prostheses are usually body powered operated by a harness and operating cord used to control a "terminal device", such as a split hook. Special devices may be required for specific tasks, e.g. a driving cup with associated ball on the steering wheel to control the motor vehicle or a snooker cue rest for pool or snooker.

If the amputation is above-elbow level an artificial elbow joint is required – in some cases these can be body powered. External power is not often used by this group of patients.

REFERENCES

Levy WS (1983) *Skin Problems of the Amputee*. Warner H. St Louis; Green Inc.

Redhead RG (1983) The early rehabilitation of lower limb amputees using a pneumatic walking aid. *Prosthet Orthot Int* 7: 88–90.

Waters RL, Perry J, Antonelli D *et al.* (1976) Energy cost of walking amputees: the influence of level of amputation. *J Bone Joint Surg* 58A: 42–46.

4.3 PAIN MANAGEMENT

S. Greenwood

VASCULAR PAIN

Despite centuries of medical interest in pain it continues to remain a complex area of management within our health care system, "*it is a source of great disability, it detracts from the quality of life and is often poorly treated*" (Moore *et al.*, 2003).

The International Association for the Study of Pain defines pain as

"*an unpleasant sensory and emotional experience associated with actual or potential tissue damage or described in terms of such damage*"

Vascular pain *per se* is a complex phenomenon experienced by many patients receiving health care treatment; it is often very distressing, chronic in nature and complicated to treat. One or more of the following produces pain of vascular disease:

1. Inadequate perfusion of tissue with resultant transient or continuous ischaemia.
2. Secondary changes, such as ulceration or gangrene.
3. Sudden or accelerated changes in the vascular wall, e.g. aneurysm.
4. Rupture of the aorta; spillage of blood will stimulate nociceptive fibres on the parietal peritoneum or pleura.
5. Intense spasm resulting from intra-arterial injection of an irritant.
6. Impairment of venous return leading to massive oedema, which stretches fascial compartments.

Can pain be harmful?

Unrelieved acute pain can have serious consequence for the individual, in both the short and long term, physiologically and psychologically.

Physiological effects may involve the respiratory, cardiovascular, gastrointestinal, neuroendocrine and metabolic systems leading to complications and delays in recovery from injury or illness.

Patients who may become frustrated with the health care system will become increasingly anxious, irritable and develop difficulty sleeping, which also will effect their recovery, this may also lead to the development of chronic pain (Macintyre & Ready, 1996; Stanik-Hunt, 1996).

The aim of acute pain management is for a pain-free patient or a patient who experiences an acceptable reduction in their pain, who is neither over sedated nor suffering side effects of analgesics.

PRINCIPLES OF PAIN MANAGEMENT

Pathophysiology of pain

There are specific nerve fibres involved in the transmission of pain messages to the brain; acute pain transmission is via A delta (Aδ) nerve fibres and chronic pain by C fibres. Aδ fibres are small diameter myelinated nerve fibres which transmit pain impulses rapidly, pain transmitted by these fibres is often described as sharp or pricking in nature and is well localised. Whereas, C fibres are unmyelinated resulting in slow transmission of impulses, pain is poorly localised and described as aching, throbbing and burning.

Cell damage occurs as a result of noxious stimuli, which may be mechanical (pressure), thermal (burn) or chemical (ischaemia) in nature.

Damaged tissues release a number of chemicals or excitatory neurotransmitters, including prostaglandins, bradykinin, serotonin (5HT), substance P and histamine, which facilitate the transduction of pain impulses along the Aδ and C nerve fibres. The non-steroidal anti-inflammatory (NSAID) group of drugs work by interfering with the production of prostaglandins, thereby assisting in reducing pain experienced by the individual.

Transduction of the pain impulse results from an action potential in the nerve fibres, which is caused by changes in the amounts of potassium and sodium ions in the neuronal membrane. Thus providing the rationale for using anti-convulsants; the process blocks or modulates sodium channels and therefore slows down the transmission of pain.

Another group of analgesic agents also work by blocking sodium channels, these are local anaesthetics which may completely stop the transmission of pain, which can be observed following nerve blocks or local infiltration of drugs, such as bupivacaine.

Transmission of pain continues with the action potential carrying the impulses from the periphery to the dorsal horn of the spinal cord, where the nociceptors terminate. From the dorsal horn the impulses pass via a number of ascending tracts (e.g. spinothalamic tract) to the brainstem and thalamus. The thalamus then relays the impulses to central structures where pain can be processed into a conscious experience.

In the dorsal horn transmission continues through the production of neurotransmitters such as adenosine, triphosphate, glutamate and substance P. It is at this site that the exogenous and endogenous opioids work by, locking on to the opioid receptors and blocking the release of the neurotransmitters, especially substance P. Pain carried by C fibres is more sensitive to opioids than that carried by the Aδ fibres. Excitatory amino acids, such as glutamate, bind to the N-methyl-D-aspirate (NMDA) receptors in the dorsal horn and facilitate the transmission of the pain impulse beyond spinal cord level.

The NMDA antagonists, which inhibit this binding of excitatory amino acids, such as ketamine, are used for pain control, however, their use has been limited due to significant side effects that can be experienced.

Debate continues around the exact central areas that are involved in the conscious experience of pain, this may be the reason for the individual differences in pain perception. Strategies such as cognitive-behavioural strategies are used which reduce the sensory and affective aspects of pain. These strategies include distraction, relaxation and imagery, distracting from the pain and reducing the number of signals transmitted to the higher centres.

Transmission of the noxious stimulus can be inhibited via tracts originating in the brainstem descending to the dorsal horn of the spinal cord, these fibres release inhibitory substances; endogenous opioids, 5HT, norepinephrine (NE), γ-aminobutyric acid (GABA) and neurotensin. Tricyclic antidepressants interfere with the reuptake of 5HT and NE, and thus increase the amounts of these substances, which provide analgesia by inhibiting the noxious stimuli (Willens, 1997; Gould & Thomas, 1997; Herbert & Paterson, 1997; Stanik-Hunt, 1997; Pasero *et al.*, 1999).

OVERVIEW OF THE ROLE OF THE PAIN CLINICAL NURSE SPECIALIST

The specialist pain nurse can provide a useful resource for the ward team to access for help when attempting to manage the pain associated with vascular disease. This type of pain can be complex, time consuming and difficult to manage for ward-based staff:

- Assessment of patients' pain.
- Recommendations for individualised treatment.
- Raise awareness of the consequences of unrelieved pain.
- Provide information and reassurance to staff, patients and their carers.
- Patient and health care professional education.
- Ensure the ward is a safe environment for pain relief techniques.
- Lead developments and advances in nursing care.
- Provide a knowledge base for multidisciplinary team to access.

Pre-operative pain management

The amount of pre-operative input required will vary according to the patients' needs: techniques/drug therapy may be initiated in this phase of the surgical process and involve input from the acute pain team (APT).

Such pain management options may or may not be required in the post-operative period; communication between the patient, ward nursing, medical, pharmacy and APTs should help to provide seamless continuity to and changes in any techniques employed.

Effective pain relief prior to surgery has been demonstrated to help reduce post-operative pain, especially in patients' undergoing limb amputation (Jensen & Nikolajsen, 1994; Weinreb, 1997; Grady & Severn, 1997; Portenoy, 1997).

All health care professionals involved have a responsibility to provide patient education, in relation to pain management it should be tailored to the individual needs of each patient and include:

- Procedural information regarding details of the medical or surgical procedure, including effects and side effects of drugs, and specialist techniques for pain management.
- Sensory information, which would describe the sensory experiences that the patient may expect, what type of pain may be experienced and how long it may last.
- Physiological coping information explains how to manage activities such as coughing and walking.

Post-operative pain management

A number of techniques can be employed to relieve post-operative pain, choice will depend on the actual surgery undertaken, the patients' overall condition pre- and post-operative, any co-existing medical conditions, concurrent drug therapy, the post-operative location of the patient, and most importantly an accurate assessment of the severity and nature of the patients pain. Techniques can be broken down into "high- and low-tech" options (Figure 4.3.1).

Epidural analgesia

In epidural analgesia low concentrations of local anaesthetics with or without opiates are infused into the epidural space via a fine bore catheter, the effect of these drugs is to provide a segmental band of analgesia around the site of surgery. The drug mixture should preferentially block the pain or sensory nerve fibres whilst avoiding a differential block of the larger nerve fibres associated with motor function, thus allowing the patient to move and walk normally. The benefits of an epidural are effective analgesia with minimal side effects and high levels of patient satisfaction. However, the choice of drugs, site of

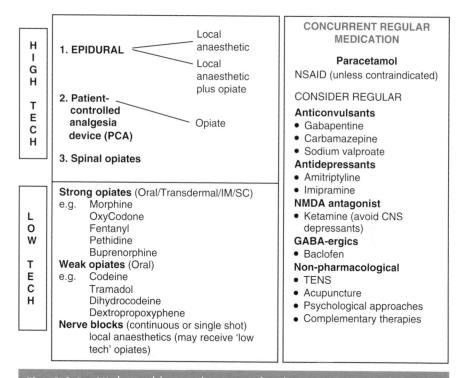

Fig. 4.3.1: High- and low-tech options for the management of post operative pain.

catheter insertion and length of duration of the technique can significantly effect the efficacy of the technique. This has to be considered along with the potential complications relating to the actual insertion of the epidural catheter (Wheatley *et al.*, 2001; Royal College of Anaesthetists, 1990). Specialist equipments (pumps) are required along with high-level observations of the patients vital signs, which require knowledgeable nursing staff.

Patient controlled analgesia

Patient controlled analgesia (PCA) allows the patient to self-administer analgesia in response to the levels of pain being experienced. The route for this technique is usually intravenous (i.v.) and uses a strong opioid such as morphine; the specialist pumps used to provide this technique have a number of safety features to avoid overdose. As with epidural infusions regular monitoring of the patients' vital signs is required, along with knowledge of the side effects of the drugs used.

Benefits of PCA

1. Avoids the peaks and troughs of analgesia and sedation associated with intramuscular (i.m.) opiate administration.

2. Self-administration puts the patient in control of the amount of pain they experience.
3. Reduces post-operative complications.
4. Reduces patient anxiety.
5. Use prophylactically to reduce procedural pain.

Adjunctive analgesia

Adjunctive analgesia should be commenced as soon as possible following surgery depending on the administration routes available, contra-indications and interactions to the drugs:

1. Paracetamol.
2. NSAIDs – reduce prostaglandin production.
3. Antidepressants.
4. Anticonvulsants.

Regular assessment of the patients' pain and any side effects is necessary, oral opiate preparations can be introduced once the patient is able to eat and drink. Such preparations often have a modified release formula to provide an "around-the-clock" effect; an immediate release preparation will also be required to cover for any episodes of "breakthrough" pain. Basic principles of pain management are detailed below:

- Individualising the regime
  - need to choose an appropriate drug,
  - choose a suitable route,
  - establish adequate dose titration, balance analgesia against side effects,
  - regular and breakthrough.
- Optimise the regime
  - schedule analgesics appropriately across a continuum of care,
  - treat procedural pain.
- Assessment which will help to identify the full nature of the pain;
- Communication with the patient, health care staff and careers;
- Multimodal analgesia improve pain relief and reduction in side effects;
- Awareness of co-existing medical diseases.

PAIN ASSESSMENT

All health care professionals have a humanitarian, moral and ethical responsibility to manage and relieve patients' pain, however, knowledge and skills are needed to facilitate this. Assessment and measurement are a crucial part of the process of pain management, requiring a systematic approach which can be repeated, involves the patient and allows for demonstration of effectiveness of interventions. In acute pain, the main types of assessment tools used are self-reporting tools:

- *Visual analogue scale (VAS)*: 10 cm line with descriptors at each end which patients are asked to mark a point on the line that best represents their pain

  No pain _____ Worst pain imaginable

- *Verbal numerical rating scale (VNRS)*: similar to VAS but the scale is broken down into 1 cm sections which are numbered, 0 = no pain to 10 = worst pain.
- *Categorical rating scale*: words are used to describe pain such as none, mild, moderate, severe, very severe and worst pain imaginable.

These three scales are easy for most patients to use and do not need special equipment to use, however, some patients find it difficult to describe their pain in such manners and the full dimensions of certain types of pain (vascular or nerve) cannot be fully explained using such scales. More extensive scales are required and often incorporate one of the former scales along with assessment of other dimensions of the pain within one extensive tool.

The pain assessment instrument described by MacCaffery and Beebe in Pain: *Clinical Manual for Nursing Practice*, is a useful tool to use and incorporates the aspects described below:

- *Intensity*: can use VAS, VNRS or categorical scale.
- *Quality*: what the pain feels like; burning, pricking, aching, throbbing, sharp.
- *Timing*: onset, duration, time intensity.
- *Impact*: upon daily activities.
- *Personal meaning*: helps with coping strategies.
- *Location*: use body chart, useful if pain radiates or more than one location.
- *Aggravating factors*: what makes the pain worse.
- *Alleviating factors*: what makes the pain better.
- *Pain behaviours*: non-verbal expressions.

PHANTOM PAIN

Phantom pain remains a puzzle for the medical profession, it has been recorded in medical literature for centuries, however, owing to the wars of the last century and developments in pain medicine it has become a recognised and accepted consequence of amputation.

Definition and classification

Phantom pain: painful sensations referred to the missing limb.
Stump pain: pain referred to the stump.
Phantom sensation: any sensation of the missing limb except pain.

Incidence

- Is reported to be between 60% and 85%.
- In certain patients (5–10%) it can become chronic persistent pain up to 2 years after amputation.
- It does not appear to be influenced by age, gender or site, or the extent of the amputation. There is evidence that severe pain prior to amputation may predispose patients to experience phantom pain.
- Phantom pain usually starts within the first week following amputation, but can occur weeks, months or years later. The pain may fluctuate in intensity, physical and emotional stimuli may increase its intensity, however, in some cases stroking the stump, applying prosthesis or applying heat can help relieve the pain. It is described as crushing, cramping, burning, stretching, knifelike or squeezing, it can be associated with spasms of the limb or stump.

Treatment

Treatment is difficult and not always successful, leading to frustration for both patients and health care professionals. There have been a number of studies over recent years but unfortunately there is no clear evidence that any one particular therapy is effective. Treatment options include:

1. Medical – drug therapies as discussed previously.
2. Surgical – e.g. dorsal column stimulation, stump revision, rhizotomy, sympathectomy.
3. Non-medical – e.g. transcutaneous electrical nerve stimulation (TENS), acupuncture, biofeedback, massage, hypnotherapy.

Most authors agree that attempts to prevent pain in the pre-operative period should be employed wherever possible, post-operatively early action is preferable, often combinations of treatment options can be used. Further research is needed to help with this complex pain phenomenon (Jensen & Nikolajsen, 1994; Weinreb, 1997; Grady & Severn, 1997; Portenoy, 1997).

REFERENCES

Gould D & Thomas VN (1997) Pain mechanisms: the neurophysiology and neuro-psychology of pain perception. In: Thomas NV (ed.). *Pain Its Nature and Management*. Bailliere Tindall, London; pp. 1–20.

Grady KM & Severn AM (1997) Post-amputation pain. In: *Key Topics in Chronic Pain*. Bios Scientific Publishers, Oxford; pp. 151–153.

Herbert LM & Paterson IS (1997) Understanding pain and its management. In: *Caring for the Vascular Patient*. Churchill Livingstone, New York; pp. 75–80.

International Association for the Study of Pain. IASP pain terminology, 1994.

Jensen TS & Nikolajsen L (1994) Phantom pain and other phenomena after amputation. In: Wall PD & Melzack R (eds). *Textbook of Pain.* Churchill Livingstone, New York; pp. 799–814.

Macintyre PE & Ready LB (1996) Acute pain: significance and assessment. In: *Acute Pain Management. A practical guide.* Saunders WB, London; pp. 1–12.

Moore A, Edwards J, Barden J & McQuay H (2003) Pain – there's a lot of it about. In: *Bandolier's Little Book of Pain.* Oxford University Press, Oxford; pp. 2–6.

Pasero C, Paice JA & MacCaffery M (1999) Basic mechanisms underlying the causes and effects of pain: In: MacCaffery M & Pasero C (eds). *Pain, Clinical Manual,* 2nd Edition. Mosby, St. Louis: pp. 15–35.

Portenoy RK (1997) Neuropathic pain. In: Kanner R (ed). *Pain Management Secrets.* Hanley & Belfus Inc., Philadelphia; pp. 122–144.

Stanik-Hunt JA (1997) Acute pain. In: Salerno E & Willens JS (eds). *Pain Management Handbook. An Interdisciplinary Approach.* Mosby, St. Louis; pp. 233–272.

The Royal College of Surgeons of England and The College of Anesthetists (1990) *Report of the Working Party on Pain After Surgery.* London.

Weinreb N (1997) Pain management in special situations. In: Salerno E & Willens JS (eds). *Pain Management Handbook. An Interdisciplinary Approach.* Mosby, St. Louis; pp. 465–523.

Wheatley RG, Schug SA & Watson D (2001) Safety and efficacy of postoperative epidural analgesia. *Br J Anaes* 87; (1): 62–73.

Willens JS (1997) Introduction to pain management. In: Salerno E & Willens JS (eds). *Pain Management Handbook. An Interdisciplinary Approach.* Mosby, St. Louis; pp. 3–38.

5

THE PERI-OPERATIVE PERIOD

5.1 THE PRE-ASSESSMENT CLINIC AND THE ROLE OF THE PRE-ASSESSMENT NURSE

L. Thompson

GENERAL AIMS OF PRE-ASSESSMENT

Pre-assessment is a service provided by some health care Trusts to patients waiting for elective surgical procedures. Its purpose is to enable health care staff to prepare patients both physically and psychologically for their forth-coming admission. By carrying out a full assessment of each individual, staff are equipped with the necessary information to identify any problems or needs likely to arise and thus deal with them prior to admission.

The pre-assessment of vascular patients is absolutely vital, as very often these patients present with co-morbidity, which place them in a high-risk category for anaesthesia. A close liaison between the pre-assessment staff and anaesthetic department is therefore essential in order to prevent last minute cancellation of these patients. This can be achieved in the following ways:

- The provision of health education may help to achieve the optimum level of fitness needed prior to surgery.
- Patients may be offered the opportunity for referral to appropriate services, such as smoking cessation, dietetics and vascular nurse specialists.
- Leaflets on health issues, such as dirt and alcohol intake, exercise tolerance and blood sugar control, can also be offered.

ROLE OF THE PRE-ASSESSMENT NURSE

The role of the pre-assessment nurse is to ensure that the aims of pre-assessment are met fully and that safe preparation of the patient for elective surgery takes place. Pre-operative assessment offers an opportunity to enhance the nursing role. The purpose of the clinic, to assess and prepare the patient means the nurse combines two roles – one previously carried out by nurses, i.e. taking a brief medical history along with social and psychological history and the other formally carried out usually by the junior doctor, who undertook the medical clerking. This merging of nursing and medical roles creates a more holistic framework.

Advantages of pre-assessment

- Patients are well prepared both physically and psychologically for their surgery.
- By following agreed protocols, patients have undergone various pre-operative investigations which enables identification of problems prior to admission.
- Patient is well informed thus aiding recovery.
- Number of patients not attending for their surgery once they have been to pre-assessment clinic is significantly reduced.
- Number of patients cancelled by the anaesthetist on the day of surgery is significantly reduced.
- Discharge planning is commenced in pre-assessment clinic thus reducing the number of delayed discharges.
- Anaesthetist has the opportunity to see the patient in the clinic if deemed necessary by the pre-assessment nurse.
- Reduction in junior doctor commitments.

Disadvantages of pre-assessment

- Anxiety may be increased by the discussion of risks of both surgery and anaesthesia. However the Patients Charter (Department of Health (DoH), 1991) states that all patients should receive clear explanations about their treatment options to help them make informed choices.
- Once the patient has been to the pre-assessment clinic, disappointment can be increased if surgery is postponed for any reason.

Vascular procedures which are pre-assessed

The vascular procedures which are pre-assessed include:
- carotid endarterectomy,
- fem pop bypass graft,
- aortic bifurcation graft for peripheral vascular disease,
- repair of abdominal aortic aneurysm,
- varicose veins.

Physical preparation of vascular patients

One of the purposes of the clinic is to assess the patients' physical suitability for an elective operation. At the clinic the nurse takes a comprehensive patient history arranging for the appropriate pre-operative tests and investigations. It is vital to gain a full assessment of the patients' general health status. Pre-assessment of vascular patients usually presents a challenge, and is rarely straightforward.

Pre-operative investigations

The pre-operative investigations will usually include:

- Full blood count (FBC).
- Urea and electrolytes (U&E).
- Clotting screen.
- Glucose/HbA1C.
- Cholesterol.
- Group and save/cross-match depending on surgery.
- Electrocardiogram (ECG).
- Chest X-ray (CXR).
- Vitalography.
- Baseline observations including blood pressure (BP) and pulse.

Psychological preparation of vascular patients

A very important aspect of pre-assessment is to prepare the patient psychologically by providing verbal and written information about the operation, the hospital episode and the expected recovery period in the ward and at home.

Of particular importance to vascular patients is the need to discuss both the risks and benefits of the operation. Discussing the risks of vascular surgery is usually quite a shock and wherever possible, written information specific to operations and conditions should be given.

The pre-assessment clinic is the ideal opportunity to provide support and counselling on a one-to-one basis away from the interruptions of a busy ward and outpatients clinic. Patients can express their fears and if necessary can be referred to a specialist vascular nurse for further discussion.

Achievement of optimum health status

This is perhaps one of the most challenging aspects of pre-assessing vascular patients. It is, first of all, necessary to assess the risk factors; a high percentage of these patients are, or have been, heavy smokers, diabetic, suffer from hypertension, raised cholesterol, ischaemic heart disease (IHD) and lead a sedentary lifestyle. Thus achieving optimum health status can be quite difficult.

Health education and advice should be offered with the availability of a wide range of leaflets and opportunity for referral to services, such as smoking cessation if available.

Patients who are diabetic should be asked to bring an up-to-date record of their glucochecks, and the need for good glycaemic control discussed.

It is also important to ensure that patients are taking their prescribed medications regularly (in particular antihypertensives, statins and aspirin) and understand the need for these medications.

Prevention of last minute cancellation

From both the patients and the surgeons point of view, this is one of the most important aspects of the pre-assessment service.

Once the results of the pre-operative tests and investigations are received, it is vital to assess them, identifying any abnormal results and act on them immediately. This is where it is important to have developed a good relationship with the anaesthetic department. It is necessary to discuss results in order to determine the next step. Often, no further action may be required other than simply making the anaesthetist aware of the patient. However, in some cases, further investigations, such as echocardiogram, may need to be arranged. If the anaesthetist feels that the patient is not physically suitable for the proposed procedure, it is better to cancel the patient prior to admission than on the day of surgery.

Commencement of discharge planning

The philosophy behind discharge planning advocates that, if possible, it should begin prior to admission. In the case of elective surgery, this is very achievable, by commencement at the pre-assessment stage.

It is necessary, firstly, to assess the patients' social circumstances, in order to identify any potential problems, and deal with them prior to admission. It is important to discuss the patients' current level of activity so that we are not setting unachievable goals. If necessary, the patient should be referred to the social work department so that they have a named social worker prior to admission and services can be arranged.

It is also important to discuss the expected length of stay so that patients can make plans prior to coming into hospital. Discharge advice sheets are also given in clinic, which inform patients what to expect when they go home, how to deal with complications and resuming normal activities, which enables patients to make any necessary arrangements.

REFERENCES

Ellen Janke, Valerie Chalk & Helen Kinley (2002) *Pre-operative Assessment, Setting a Standard Through Learning*, by Ellen Janke, University of Southampton, Southampton, UK.

5.2   VASCULAR ANAESTHESIA

A. Shakir

The advances in surgery and anaesthesia have made surgery of the aorta and its major branches a common occurrence in modern operation theatres. In a typical District General Hospital, vascular surgery comprises of operations on infra-renal aortic reconstruction, carotid endarterectomy and lower limb revascularisation.

THE VASCULAR PATIENT

Pre-operative assessment of patients involves a full history, examination and investigation for preparation for surgical procedures. These patients are usually Grade III on American Society of Anaesthesiologists (ASA) and require high-dependency unit/intensive care unit (HDU/ICU) especially following aortic surgery.

The functions that affect mortality in vascular surgery are as follows:

1. Emergency surgery carries a high mortality rate up to 50–80% with ruptured aortic aneurysms. Elective surgery has a 10% mortality rate.
2. Age and sex of patients. The majority of patients are males between 60- and 80-year old, with peripheral vascular disease more prevalent in males.
3. The prevalence of co-existing disease in patients for vascular surgery:
   – Hypertension (40–60%): The effect on cardiovascular health is widespread. It accelerates the artherosclerotic process. Mortality is directly related to the involvement of major target organs, e.g. the brain, the heart and the kidney. Hypertension causes ventricular hypertrophy and an increase in the risk of myocardial infarction and cardiac failure, stroke, aortic dissection and ruptured aortic aneurysm, as well as sudden death.
   The widespread increase in arteriolar resistance causes reduction in the intravascular volume and exaggerated responses to the anaesthetic agent in the form of hypotension, and hypertension to light anaesthetic.
   – Heart disease (50–70%): It is very common for those requiring aortic surgery to suffer from ischaemic heart disease (IHD) and have the symptoms of angina (10–20%), a history of previous myocardial infarction (40–60%) or congestive heart failure (5–15%).
   Pre-operative assessment is essential in establishing the degree of coronary artery disease or previous myocardial infarction. There is

significant risk of infarction in the peri-operative period. Procedures should be postponed by 6 months following a myocardial infarction to reduce the risk of reinfarction to only 4–5%.

Anaesthesia in patients with congestive cardiac failure can increase the risk of hypoxia, reduce cardiac output, overt pulmonary oedema, hypotension and malignant dysrhythmia.

– Renal disease (5–25%): Renal damage due to hypertension, congestive cardiac failure and involvement of the renal arteries in atherosclerotic, and aneurysmal disease will lead to a degree of renal failure reflected in increased pre-operative plasma concentrations of urea and creatine. Vascular surgery may be associated with sudden haemorrhage and temporary mechanical occlusion of renal vessels. This causes acute tubular necrosis and renal failure.

– Chronic obstructive pulmonary disease (COPD) (25–50%): Many patients with vascular disease are (or were) heavy smokers with significant COPD. Normally abdominal surgery leads to reduced lung volumes, with shallow tidal volumes, reduced or absent sighing, weakened cough and impaired gas exchange. Patients with COPD are at higher risk of developing post-operative pulmonary complications.

Pre-operative preparations are therefore required with physiotherapy, bronchodilators and cessation of smoking to significantly reduce the risk of these complications.

– Diabetes (8–12%): This group of patients suffer with a high incidence of peripheral vascular disease that requires revascularisation or amputation, especially when the perfusion is inadequate leading to tissue breakdown, sore and infection pre-operatively.

Management of diabetes pre-operatively consists of management of blood glucose levels with intravenous (i.v.) glucose and insulin sliding scales.

Patients on oral antidiabetic medication should stop 24 h pre-operatively and should instead have insulin administered intravenously.

CAROTIDENDARTERECTOMY

From the anaesthetic point of view, this operation on the extracranial portion of the carotid artery involves:

1. *Surgery near the airway*: The airway needs to be reliably secured during the operation, especially if general anaesthetic is being used. There needs to be careful positioning with moderate cervical extension and rotation away from the site of operation. Avoid venous obstruction and straining the cervical spine, especially if the patient has cervical spondylosis.

2. *Temporary occlusion*: Temporary occlusion due to clamping of the carotid artery on the affected side leads the brain to depend on collateral flow via the Circle of Willis to maintain cerebral oxygen supply.

Assessment
- Full medical, history and anaesthetic examination.
- Investigations should include full blood count (FBC), urea and electrolytes (U&E), blood glucose, electrocardiogram (ECG), chest X-ray (CXR), respiratory function test and echocardiogram when indicated in order to optimise general condition and effective treatment of co-existing diseases.
- Explaining the anaesthetic management plan often reduces patient anxiety. Premedication is routinely offered which is an anxiolytic drug if required.
- Patients are advised to continue with cardiac medication on the day of the operation.

Anaesthetic technique
1. *General anaesthesia*: General anaesthesia with controlled ventilation to provide stable cardiovascular conditions, avoiding myocardial infarction or cerebral ischaemia.
   - *Anaesthesia*: In the anaesthetic room, oxygen is supplied to the patient with a face mask. Full monitoring is also required, with an ECG, pulse oximeter, direct blood pressure (BP) measurement with an intra-arterial cannula. Use peripheral veins to adequately hydrate the patient using Hartman's solution or normal saline and avoid using dextrose solution. Hyperglycaemia worsens a cerebral ischaemia in the peri-operative period.
   - *Induction*: The aim is to maintain cardiovascular stability, thiopentone or propofol with muscle relaxant and endotrachial tube. Preformed Rae tubes are ideal to allow easy connection with ventilator tubing. The patient's eyes should be protected. Total intravenous anaesthesia (TIVA) can also be used.
   - *Maintenance*: Balanced anaesthesia, analgesia and muscle relaxant should be used to aim for normocapnia and stable BP. There should be continuous monitoring of the ECG, especially the ST-segment for the detection of sub-endocardial ischaemia and bradydysrhythmias which can be caused by dissection around the carotid sinus nerve. This can be blocked by infiltration of lignocaine.
   Monitoring of BP should aim for a systolic BP of ± 40 mmHg of the patient's baseline systolic BP.
   Fraction of inspired oxygen (F_iO_2) is to be maintained at 50%. Arterial oxygen saturation (S_aO_2) and capnography should also be monitored.
   Heparinisation (3000–5000 units) is required before clamping the artery.

2. *Local anaesthesia*: Cervical epidural or selectively blocking (on the operation side) the ventral branch of the cervical nerve roots C2, C3 and C4 local infiltration of the skin especially at the lower part of the neck is desirable because of innervation of the skin from the opposite side. This technique provides immediate and continuous monitoring of the collateral cerebral circulation. The patient becomes drowsy if the blood supply to the brain is inadequate which then requires the use of a shunt.

Post-operative management

- The anaesthetic technique should allow for rapid recovery for neurological assessment.
- Haemodynamic stability is also important. Maintain BP with normal ranges and treat hyper/hypotension with vasopressors or vasodilators and if required, to maintain patients baseline systolic BP to ±40 mmHg.
- Discharge for recovery after a reasonable period of observation (approximately 2–3 h).
- Subsequent observation in HDU for 12–24 h.

Reported post-operative complications

1. Haemodynamic instability.
2. Airway obstruction.
3. Vocal cord palsy due to recurrent laryngeal nerve damage.
4. Neurological deficits following surgery due to plaque fragmentation and mobilisation.
5. Chemoreceptor dysfunction due to bilateral dysfunction that results in complete loss of hypoxic drive.

ABDOMINAL AORTIC SURGERY

A major surgical procedure on usually high-risk patients for aneurysmal dilatation (which might rupture suddenly) or atherosclerotic occlusion of the aorta and major branches which causes leg pain (claudication).

Intra-operative haemodynamic and ischaemic complications are mainly caused by cross clamping that is necessary to insert the graft across the diseased segment of the aorta.

The main post-operative complication is myocardial infarction.

Assessment

- Aim for a selection of suitable patients for the surgery to improve outcomes. Also aim to optimise general conditions by treating co-existing diseases.

- Full medical, anaesthetic history, examination and investigations should include the following: FBC, U&E, 12-lead ECG, CXR, respiratory function test, echocardiography.
- Further tests may be indicated, e.g.: exercise and/or ambulatory 24 h ECG, stress echocardiography, radionuclide scanning.
- Significant coronary artery disease needs to be revascularised before carrying out vascular surgery. The same also applies to significant carotid artery disease.
- ICU/HDU beds need to be booked for post-operative management of these patients.

Premedications

The anaesthetic visit explains the anaesthetic management to the patient. It often relieves their anxiety, however sometimes premedications are required, such as temazepam.

The patient should continue cardiac medication even on the day of operation.

Anaesthetic room

1. Institute monitoring.
2. ECG.
3. Pulse oximeter.
4. Central venous pressure (CVP) catheter or pulmonary artery catheter.
5. Epidural catheter (thoracic).

Induction

1. Pre-oxygenation.
2. General anaesthesia aiming at haemodynamic stability at induction and intubation.
3. Insertion of nasogastric tube.
4. Insertion of urinary catheter.

Maintenance

The patient should be supine with both arms out for ease of access. Balanced anaesthesia with invasive positive pressure ventilation (IPPV) should be aiming for cardiovascular stability.

Intra-operative monitoring includes: ECG lead II and V5 ST-segment analysis, S_aO_2, capnography, F_iO_2, core temperature monitoring, direct BP, CVP, urine output.

Special requirement for aortic surgery

1. *Heparin* (5000 units) is required prior to cross clamping.

2. *Cross-clamping* of the aorta produces a marked increase in left ventricular afterload in patients with aneurysmal disease.

   This response does not occur in patients with occlusive disease due to the gradual narrowing of the aorta, iliac arteries and the development of collateral circulation.

   An i.v. infusion of vasodilator, the use of volatile anaesthetic or epidural sympathetic blockade can all reduce the effects of this sudden increase in ventricular afterload.

3. Furthermore, an *aortic cross-clamping* release may cause severe hypotension. Prior volume load and controlled release of the cross clamp by the surgeon with the use of vasopressors will ensure adequate venous return and adequate coronary perfusion.

4. *Blood replacement.* Normally 6 units of blood should be cross-matched. An average of 4 units of blood is required for transfusion. Fresh frozen plasma (FFP) needs to be transfused if further blood is required.

EMERGENCY ABDOMINAL AORTIC SURGERY

Patient may present either with a leaking aneurysm and stable haemodynamic profile or a ruptured aneurysm with unstable haemodynamic profile, which is fatal if untreated urgently.

Pre-operative management
- Formal assessment and investigation are rarely possible.
- Large gauge i.v. cannula should be inserted preferably more than one.
- Blood is immediately sent for cross-matching (10–12 units). O negative blood may be used if cross-matched blood is not available or is delayed.
- Crystalloid, colloid, blood and blood products should be infused with a blood warmer and rapid infusion pump to maintain recordable BP around 80 mmHg.
- When the surgeon and theatre staff are ready, induction of anaesthesia should start (when the surgeon is ready to make skin incision). Minimal doses of induction agent should be used, with rapid sequence induction technique. Hypotension is anticipated, as abdominal tamponade effect is lost.

Maintenance
- Balanced anaesthesia with 100% oxygen and opiate (remifentanil) infusion with small boluses of midazolam and/or volatile anaesthetic to prevent awareness.
- Insertion of CVP, arterial line, urinary catheter and nasogastric tube is required.
- The surgical priority is to control bleeding by cross clamping the aorta.

- Monitoring include ECG, S_aO_2, F_iO_2, capnography, invasive arterial pressure, CVP, core temperature and urine output.

Special points

- Large volume of blood loss which need to be replaced will result in dilutional coagulopathy. FFP and platelets transfusion will be required guided by coagulation study.
- Controlled cross-clamp release by the surgeon to avoid severe hypotension.

Post-operative management

- Transfer to intensive therapy unit (ITU) with IPPV continued until stable cardiovascular and respiratory functions are achieved.
- Aiming at normal oxygen-carrying capacity, normothermia and correction of coagulation defect.
- Recognition and treatment of complications, such as bleeding from the site of surgery, limb ischaemia, gastrointestinal and spinal cord ischaemia, myocardial infarction, respiratory and renal failures.
- Good analgesia (epidural) will facilitate early extubation and ambulation.

Outcome

- The mortality in emergency aortic surgery 50–80%.
- Patient selection significantly influence outcome.

When there is no real hope of survival, surgery should not be carried out, and these patients should be provided with good analgesia and nursing care.

REVASCULARISATION OF THE LOWER LIMBS

Lower limbs atherosclerosis is common in elderly patients, particularly those with a long history of smoking.

They present to surgery for either of the following:

- *Acute ischaemia* due to embolic event which then requires femoral embolectomy under local anaesthesia.
- *Chronic ischaemia* due to atherosclerosis which requires a bypass graft, to improve the blood flow to the distal region. The bypass operation depends on the site of obstruction.

Assessment

- Medical and anaesthetic history, examination and full investigations, e.g. FBC, U&E, ECG, CXR and respiratory function test.

- The aim is to optimise general condition and treatment of co-existing disease, e.g. hypertension, diabetes, congestive cardiac failure, etc.
- To plan anaesthetic management and the provision of post-operative analgesia.

Premedication

Explain anaesthetic management to the patient and offer premedication, if required prescribe anxiolytic drug. No premedication required in patient who is already obtunded.

Advise to continue with cardiac medication.

Anaesthetic technique

The aim is to provide haemodynamic stability. The choice of the technique will depend on the experience, patient conditions and length of surgery. The options are general anaesthesia, or regional anaesthesia (spinal or epidural) or combined general and nerve block. Other factors that influence the choice is the severity of pre-existing cardiovascular or respiratory disease.

Monitoring during anaesthesia

The standard monitoring.

Post-operative management

Observation in recovery room until the patient is stable and provision of adequate analgesia.

Oxygen via face mask for 3 days in poor risk patients or when patient-controlled analgesia (PCA) is prescribed.

FURTHER READING

Caldicott L, Lumb A & McCoy D "*Vascular Anaesthesia: A Practical Handbook*".

Cunningham AJ (1989) "Anaesthesia for abdominal aortic surgery: a review (Part 1)" *Can J Anaesth* 36: 426–444.

Foex P & Reeder MK (1993) Anaesthesia for vascular surgery. *Clin Anaesthesiol* 7: 97–126.

Joel A, Kaplan & Carol L (1991) Lake (eds) *Vascular Anesthesia*. Churchill Livingstone, New York.

5.3 OPERATIVE VASCULAR SURGERY: COMMON VASCULAR OPERATIONS

O. Ehsan and H. Al-Khaffaf

CAROTID ENDARTERECTOMY

Indications

The indication for carotid endarterectomy is a combination of high-grade carotid artery stenosis (>70%) with significant symptoms. The symptoms include transient ischaemic attacks (TIAs), amaurosis fugax, retinal infarction and non-disabling stroke.

Assessment

- Careful history and examination.
- The investigations used to determine carotid artery stenosis include Duplex ultrasound, arteriography, computerised tomography (CT) angiography or magnetic resonance imaging.
- Once the decision of operation is made, the general fitness of the patient is assessed. This will include checking the cardiac, pulmonary and renal functions.
- Informed consent should be obtained highlighting the benefits and risks of the procedure.

Operative technique

Carotid endarterectomy can be performed under local or general anaesthesia. The advantage of local anaesthesia is that the patient's mental status can be assessed all the time and no other cerebral monitoring is required. Intra-operative shunt can be used with early recognition of changes in the level of consciousness or motor deficits and the risk of a peri-operative stroke is minimised.

A vertical incision is made along the anterior border of sternocleidomastoid muscle and dissection is carefully carried down to the carotid sheath.

The carotid bifurcation is then identified and adequate proximal and distal exposure is obtained to allow for clamping above and below the plaque.

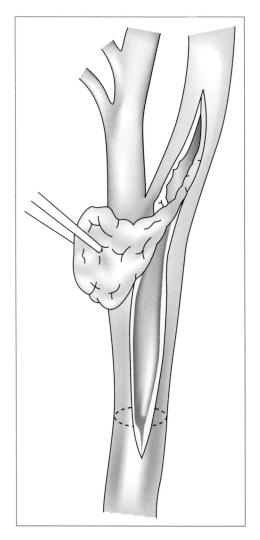

Fig. 5.3.1: Carotid endarterectomy, the plaque being dissected from the carotid bifurcation.

The patient is then heparinised and clamps are applied to the common, internal and external carotid arteries. A longitudinal arteriotomy is made over internal carotid and common carotid arteries, and the plaque is displayed.

Endarterectomy is then carried out by dissecting the plaque off the arterial wall carefully, especially at the distal end of the internal carotid artery to avoid intimal dissection (Figure 5.3.1).

When the procedure is performed under general anaesthesia, some surgeons use an indwelling shunt routinely to minimise the risk of stroke. Others are guided by the changes displayed by a transcranial Doppler.

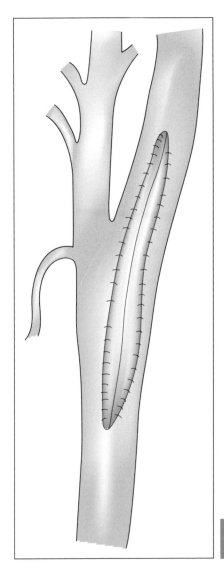

Fig. 5.3.2: Closure of the arteriotomy with a patch.

The arteriotomy may then be closed primarily with a non-absorbable suture or with a vein or prosthetic patch. The repair is then checked for leaks and a suction drain may be used. Closure is done in layers (Figures 5.3.2 and 5.3.3).

Complications

The major complications are:

1. Haemorrhage due to either a leak from the anastomosis or bleeding from wound itself.

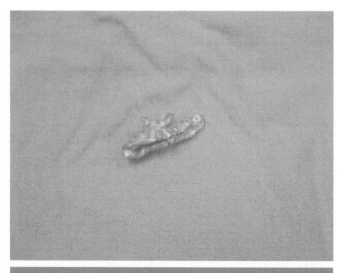

Fig. 5.3.3: A removed carotid plaque.

2. Stroke which can be either immediate or post-operative (within 24 h).
3. Peri-operative myocardial infarction.
4. Partial or complete cranial nerve injury (vagus, hypoglossal, glossopharyngeal, recurrent laryngeal).

ABDOMINAL AORTIC ANEURYSM REPAIR

Indications
Surgery for abdominal aortic aneurysm may be done as an emergency or as an elective procedure. The aneurysm may be infra-renal (>90% of cases) or supra-renal.

- *Emergency*: Around 50% patients with rupture survive to reach the hospital. This may be an anterior rupture or posterior rupture (better survival).
- *Elective*: Electively the procedure may be done in a symptomatic patient (abdominal or back pain) or an asymptomatic patient with aneurysm diameter >5.5 cm on ultrasound.

Assessment
- Assessment of the size of the aneurysm is done with ultrasonography. A CT scan is used to determine the relationship of the aneurysm to the renal and iliac arteries.
- The pre-operative assessment includes checking the cardiac, pulmonary and renal functions of the patient. This will include full blood count with

grouping and cross matching, electrolytes, urea and creatinine, liver function tests, electrocardiogram, chest radiograph, pulmonary function test and echocardiography.

- Informed consent should be obtained highlighting the benefits and risks of the operation.

Operative technique

The patient is catheterised and operation is done under general anaesthesia. Central venous and arterial lines are also passed for monitoring.

A midline or upper transverse abdominal incision can be used. The small intestine is packed to the right and abdominal aorta is identified.

In case of emergency surgery, a clamp is immediately placed above the proximal extent of aneurysm. Occasionally supra-renal clamping may be required.

In elective cases, the posterior peritoneum is opened and renal vessels are identified. Iliac arteries are dissected and heparin is given. Proximal and distal clamps are placed above and below the aneurysm sac after palpation to identify the condition of the vessel.

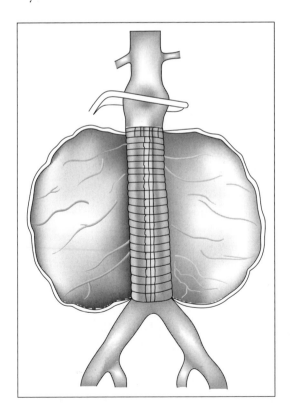

Fig. 5.3.4: A straight tube graft is used if the aneurysm does not involve the iliac arteries.

The aneurysm is opened longitudinally and debris from the sac evacuated. Back bleeding from lumbar vessels is controlled with sutures placed from inside the sac. Inferior mesenteric artery may be ligated at this stage.

The graft is then sutured end-to-end inside the aneurysm sac (inlay technique), proximal end first and followed by the distal end. The upper anastomosis is tested before doing the lower one (Figures 5.3.4 and 5.3.5).

Clamps on iliac arteries are released one at a time. The aneurysm sac is then closed over the graft and posterior peritoneum is closed. A drain may be used in the retroperitoneal space and the abdomen is closed in layers.

Occasionally the iliac vessels can be involved in the aneurysm and then an aortic bifurcation graft can be used either into the iliac arteries (aorto-bi-iliac) or into the femoral arteries (aorto-bi-femoral) (Figure 5.3.6).

Complications
The major complications are:

1. Myocardial infarction.
2. Renal failure which may be due to hypotension or supra-renal clamping of aorta.
3. Respiratory complications (pneumonia and respiratory failure).

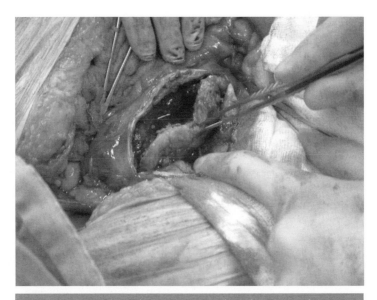

Fig. 5.3.5: A thrombus is seen within the opened aneurysm sac.

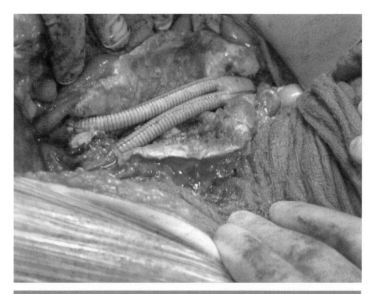

Fig. 5.3.6: In this case the aneurysm involved the iliac arteries and therefore the repair required a bifurcated graft between the aorta and the iliac arteries.

4. Ischaemic colitis.
5. Spinal cord ischaemia.

THORACO-ABDOMINAL ANEURYSM REPAIR

Indications

A thoraco-abdominal aneurysm >5 cm in diameter is an indication for surgery because the risk of rupture is significantly high.

Thoraco-abdominal aneurysms involve a segment of aorta from which coeliac axis, superior and inferior mesenteric arteries and renal arteries arise. Surgical repair of these aneurysms has a higher risk of ischaemic damage to spinal cord, kidneys and intestine, and later development of multiple organ failure.

Assessment

- Repair of these aneurysms is a major undertaking and is usually performed in a few centres in the UK.
- Careful assessment of the patient fitness is therefore essential. This includes cardiac, respiratory and renal functions.
- Informed consent is taken, explaining the risks and benefits.

Operative technique

The operative exposure requires a large oblique thoraco-abdominal incision through sixth or seventh intercostals space and going below the umbilicus.

The diaphragm is divided along the periphery. The descending thoracic aorta is identified in the left chest and the proximal end of aneurysm is isolated.

The retroperitoneum is opened to expose the abdominal aorta and its bifurcation. The patient is heparinised and the aorta is clamped proximally in the chest.

The distal aorta may be left open or clamped and perfused. The aneurysm is incised and proximal anastomosis between aorta and graft is performed.

The abdominal visceral and intercostals arteries are re-implanted into the graft. Finally the distal anastomosis is performed between the graft and distal aorta.

Complications

The major complications are:

1. Paraplegia due to spinal cord ischaemia.
2. Acute renal failure.
3. Respiratory complications.
4. Intestinal ischaemia.
5. Multiple organ failure.
6. Bleeding.

PROCEDURES USED FOR REVASCULARISATION OF THE LOWER LIMBS

Aorto-bi-femoral bypass for occlusive disease

Indications

Indications for aorto-femoral or aorto-bi-femoral bypass for occlusive disease are:

1. Critical ischaemia or threatened limb loss with rest pain.
2. Ulceration.
3. Gangrene.
4. Atheroembolic phenomena (blue toe syndrome).
5. Disabling claudication sufficient enough to impair lifestyle (following failure of balloon angioplasty).

Assessment

- A careful history and examination followed by detailed assessment is required. Assessment of the occlusive disease is done with Duplex ultrasonography, arteriography or CT angiogram. Magnetic resonance angiography is non-invasive and gives anatomical picture of the disease.

- The pre-operative assessment includes checking the cardiac, pulmonary and renal status of the patient. This will include full blood count with grouping and cross matching, electrolytes, urea and creatinine, liver function tests, electrocardiogram, chest radiograph and pulmonary function test.
- Informed consent should be obtained.

Operative technique

Midline or transverse abdominal incision can be used to reach the lower aorta and bifurcation. Similarly groin incision can be longitudinal or skin crease.

The retroperitoneum is opened and the site of proximal anastomosis on aorta is selected. In the groin common femoral artery is dissected out at the level of division into superficial femoral and profunda femoris.

Patient is heparinised, and proximal and distal control is obtained at both the ends.

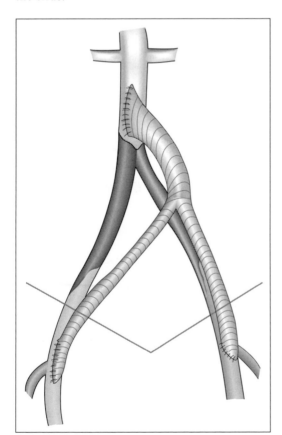

Fig. 5.3.7: An aorto-bi-femoral bypass should only be considered if the limb is critically ischaemic and after failure of balloon angioplasty.

The proximal anastomosis of bifurcation graft with aorta can be done in an end-to-end or end-to-side manner. The graft limb is then passed through a tunnel created over the external iliac vessels, taking care that it does not twist.

The distal anastomosis is done in an end-to-side fashion between graft and common femoral artery at the level of its division. The anastomosis is tested and then the limb perfusion is checked. Sometimes an embolectomy may be required to remove any thrombus or embolus in the distal vessel. Suction drains are placed and closure is done in layers (Figure 5.3.7).

Complications

The major complications are:

1. Haemorrhage.
2. Myocardial infarction.
3. Respiratory complications.
4. Thrombosis of graft.
5. Trash foot (distal embolisation of ateromatous material).
6. Ischaemia of distal large intestine.
7. Graft infection.
8. Sexual dysfunction (retrograde ejaculation or impotence).

Femoro-popliteal bypass grafts

Indications
Indications for femoro-popliteal bypass graft include:

1. Severe disabling claudication.
2. Limb-threatening critical ischaemia or rest pain.
3. Gangrene.
4. Non-healing arterial ulcers.

Assessment
- Careful history about claudication distance, rest pain, colour changes, numbness, parasthesia, motor or sensory loss, ulceration and gangrene is taken. This is followed by careful physical examination of temperature, capillary fill, pulses, sensation, ulcer or gangrene.
- Assessment of the occlusive disease is done with Duplex ultrasonography followed by arteriography for anatomical picture. Magnetic resonance angiography is non-invasive and can be used.

Operative technique
Transverse or vertical incision can be used in the groin and a vertical incision is made above or below the knee.

Graft is bridged between common femoral artery in the groin and popliteal artery above or below the knee. Graft choices are autogenous vein or prosthetic graft materials (expanded polytetrafluoroethylene (ePTFE), Dacron). The venous graft is preferred and may be used as a reversed bypass or/and *in situ* bypass with disruption of valves.

The incisions are made, and common femoral and popliteal arteries are exposed. Proximal and distal control is obtained. Patient is heparinised and vessels clamped.

If a prosthetic graft is being used then tunnelling device is used to pass it subcutaneously. The proximal and distal anastomosis is then made, in an end-to-side manner, between the graft and common femoral artery proximally and popliteal artery distally using 5/0 or 6/0 prolene. The anastomosis is tested and then the limb perfusion is checked (Figure 5.3.8).

Suction drains may be placed and closure is done in layers.

Complications
The complications include:

1. Haemorrhage.
2. Wound infection.
3. Failure/thrombosis of graft.
4. Trash foot (distal embolisation of atheromatous material).
5. Lymphatic leak from the groin wound due to lymphatic damage.

Femoro-tibial bypass grafts
Indications
The indications for femoro-tibial/distal bypass are the same as those for femoro-popliteal bypass. However, in these cases the popliteal artery cannot be used due to its involvement in disease process.

Assessment
- Careful history about claudication distance, rest pain, colour changes, numbness, parasthesia, motor or sensory loss, ulceration and gangrene is taken. This is followed by careful physical examination of temperature, capillary fill, pulses, sensation, ulcer or gangrene.
- Assessment of the occlusive disease is done with duplex ultrasonography followed by arteriography for anatomical assessment. Magnetic resonance angiography is non-invasive and can be used.
- Informed consent should be obtained.

Operative technique

Transverse or vertical incision can be used in the groin. A vertical incision is made medially below the knee the level of which depends on the patent distal artery being considered for anastomosis. The graft is bridged between the common femoral artery and the tibial arteries.

Autogenous vein is the graft of choice as it has a much better patency than prosthetic grafts (ePTFE, Dacron). However, the use of an interposition venous cuff or patch between the graft and the distal artery has been shown to improve the patency of prosthetic grafts. In the case of an *in situ* technique the long saphenous vein is used.

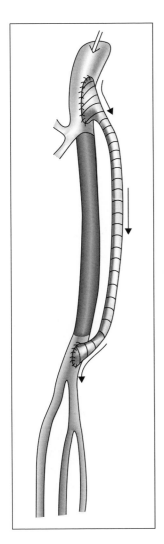

Fig. 5.3.8: Reversed long saphenous vein is the preferred graft for femoro-popliteal bypasses.

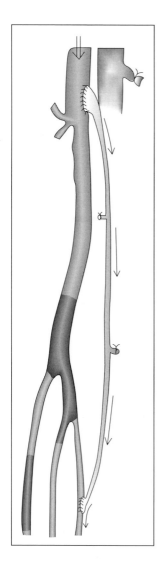

Fig. 5.3.9: Femoro-tibial bypass.

The incisions are made and common femoral and tibial arteries are exposed. Proximal and distal control is obtained. The patient is heparinised and vessels are clamped.

If a prosthetic graft is being used then a tunnelling device is used to pass it subcutaneously. The proximal and distal anastomosis is then made, in an end-to-side manner, between the graft and common femoral artery proximally and tibial artery distally using 5/0 or 6/0 prolene. The anastomosis is tested and then the limb perfusion is checked.

Suction drains may be placed and closure is done in layers (Figure 5.3.9).

Complications

The complications include:

1. Haemorrhage.
2. Infection.
3. Failure/thrombosis of graft.
4. Trash foot (distal embolisation of atheromatous material).

Profundoplasty

Indications

This procedure is indicated in the cases of stenosis or occlusion of the profunda femoris artery at its origin from common femoral artery.

Operative technique

Transverse or vertical groin incision is used. The common femoral artery and its branches are exposed. Intravenous heparin is given and clamps are applied.

An incision is made into the common femoral artery and extended down into the profunda femoris artery. Endarterectomy of the profunda is then carried out (Figures 5.3.10 and 5.3.11).

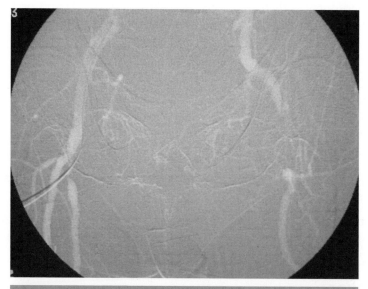

Fig. 5.3.10: An angiogram showing an occlusion of the left common and superficial femoral arteries as well as the origin of the profunda femoris.

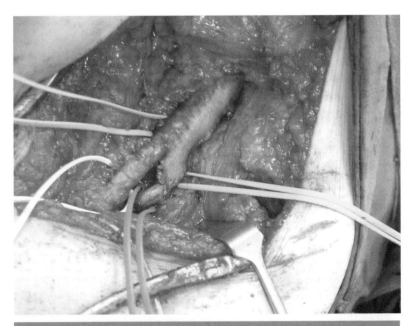

Fig. 5.3.11: Endarterectomy and patch profundoplasty in the same patient in Figure 5.3.9.

This arteriotomy is then closed using a patch of vein, Dacron or PTFE to widen the narrowed segment. The wound is then closed in layers.

Complications

The complications are:

1. Haemorrhage.
2. Infection.
3. Re-stenosis.

Extra-anatomical bypass procedures for aorto-iliac occlusive disease

Extra-anatomic revascularisation procedures include axillo-femoral bypass and cross over femoro-femoral bypass to get the arterial flow from upper extremity or the opposite femoral artery.

Indications

1. Patients who are unfit for major abdominal procedure.
2. Lower extremity ischaemia in the presence of an infected aortic graft.
3. Re-operation for aorto-femoral graft occlusion.

Axillo-femoral bypass

Operative technique

Infra-clavicular incision is made to expose the proximal axillary artery.

A vertical incision is made in the groin to expose the common femoral artery at the level of its bifurcation. Prosthetic graft materials are always used.

The graft is tunnelled subcutaneously along the lateral aspect of the trunk. Anastomosis is done end-to-side, to the ipsilateral femoral artery in case of axillo-unifemoral bypass or to both femoral arteries for axillo-bifemoral bypass.

These patients with a long prosthetic graft are usually anticoagulated post-operatively to prevent graft thrombosis.

Cross over femoro-femoral bypass

Operative technique

A patent donor iliac artery is required. Both femoral arteries are exposed by vertical incisions in the groin. The graft is tunnelled subcutaneously in the supra-pubic region and end-to-side anastomosis is made between the graft and both femoral arteries using 5/0 or 6/0 prolene.

Cross over femoro-femoral bypass has better patency rate than the axillo-femoral bypass.

Complications

The complications are:

1. Haemorrhage.
2. Infection.
3. Failure/thrombosis of graft causing distal ischaemia or gangrene.

REPAIR OF POPLITEAL ANEURYSMS

A popliteal aneurysm is the most common peripheral aneurysm and can accompany aortic aneurysm. It can present as a swelling behind the knee or with complications of distal ischaemia due to thrombosis or embolism (Figures 5.3.12 and 5.3.13).

Physical examination reveals a pulsatile swelling in the popliteal fossa. This can be confirmed with an ultrasound or CT scan.

Due to the risk of complications some surgeons tend to repair these aneurysms irrespective of the size or symptoms. However, the consensus is

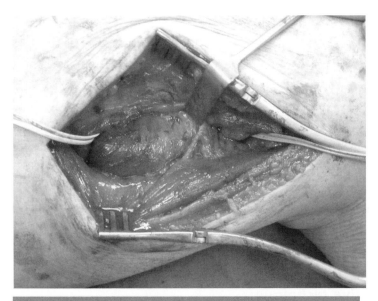

Fig. 5.3.12: A large popliteal aneurysm.

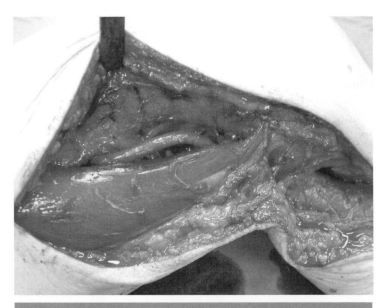

Fig. 5.3.13: The long saphenous vein was used to bypass the popliteal aneurysm in the same patient in Figure 5.3.11.

that these aneurysms should be treated if they are symptomatic or measure >3 cm in diameter.

The repair is usually surgical. This can be either via a posterior incision with excision of the aneurysm and interposition graft or inlay graft, or a medial incision with ligation of the aneurysm and bypass around the popliteal space with a vein graft.

ENDOSCOPIC THORACIC SYMPATHECTOMY

Indications
1. Hyperhydrosis of the palms. Isolated axillary sweating should be treated by Botox injection rather than sympathectomy.
2. Facial blushing and sweating.

Assessment
- As the main indication for this procedure is a social problem, it is extremely important that the patient is well informed about the benefits and the complications of this operation. Failure to do so may result in a considerable dissatisfaction by the patient.
- As the majority of these patients are aged <30, no special investigations are required pre-operatively. A chest X-ray is routinely done to exclude any pulmonary pathology.

Operative technique
This is done using a suitable endoscope. Two ports are usually used, one for the camera, and the other for dissection and coagulation.

The pleural cavity can be filled with CO_2 and the lung is simply deflated using a double lumen tube. The trocars are placed in the third and fourth intercostals spaces between mid-clavicular line and mid-axillary line.

After passing the endoscope, the sympathetic chain is identified as a shiny cord running on the neck of the ribs and is dissected out from behind the pleura (Figure 5.3.14).

A coagulating electrode is then used to destroy the sympathetic ganglia. Haemostasis is secured and all the gas is sucked out while inflating the lung. The insertion sites are then closed.

Post-operative chest X-ray is done to check for proper lung inflation. A chest tube may be required if there is a significant residual pneumothorax.

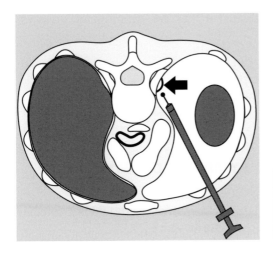

Fig. 5.3.14: A diagram demonstrating the position of the endoscope and the sympathetic chain.

Complications

The major complications are:

1. Compensatory truncal sweating.
2. Gustatory sweating (sweating on eating hot or spicy food).
3. Pneumothorax.
4. Injury to surrounding structures.
5. Injury to stellate ganglion producing Horner's syndrome.
6. Recurrence due to incomplete procedure.

VARICOSE VEINS

Indications

Surgery for varicose veins, involving long or short saphenous system in the lower limb, is considered when they are symptomatic or present with complications.

Assessment

- The assessment of patients should be done clinically to determine the incompetence in the superficial system and to rule out incompetence of deep venous system.
- This may be followed by investigations, like venous Duplex studies or venography, for the deep system.
- When the decision for surgery is made then the patient is assessed regarding fitness for surgery.

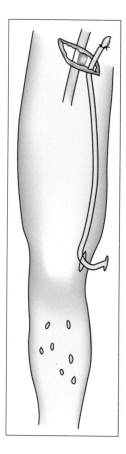

Fig. 5.3.15: The principle of varicose vein surgery involves sapheno-femoral junction ligation, stripping of the long saphenous vein and multiple avulsions.

Operation
Operative technique for varicose veins affecting long saphenous system

The operation for varicose veins for long saphenous system comprises of:

- High ligation of long saphenous vein at its junction with the femoral vein.
- Stripping of long saphenous vein.
- Multiple avulsions of the superficial varices.

Pre-operatively the varices are marked with skin marker.

Initially an oblique incision is made in the inguinal skin crease medial to the palpable femoral pulsations.

The junction between the long saphenous vein and the femoral vein is dissected out. All the tributaries draining into the saphenous vein are ligated and cut and the long saphenous vein is then ligated at its junction with the femoral vein and divided (Figure 5.3.15).

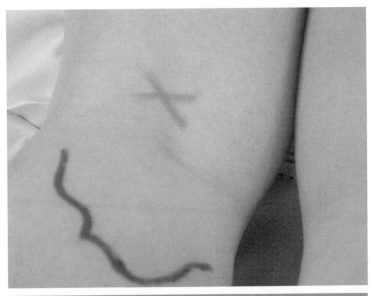

Fig. 5.3.16: The position of the sapheno-popliteal junction has been marked with an (X) preoperatively by Duplex scan.

A stripper is passed into the distal end of long saphenous vein until it is palpable around the level of the knee. It is identified and retrieved through a small transverse incision. Stripping below the level of knee joint may cause damage of the saphenous nerve. The whole length of the vein is examined after it is stripped.

For multiple avulsions small (1–2 mm) stab incisions are made over the marked sites and the superficial varices are hooked out and avulsed. The inguinal incision is closed with sub-cuticular skin stitch. The small stab incisions may be closed by skin adhesive strips or clips.

Post-operative dressing consists of compression bandage which is changed, before discharge, to compression stockings for 2 weeks.

Operative technique for sapheno-popliteal junction ligation
The operation for varicose veins for short saphenous system comprises of:

- ligation of short saphenous vein at its junction with the popliteal vein;
- multiple avulsions of the superficial varices;

Pre-operatively the sapheno-popliteal junction needs to be marked by Duplex scan as it may be very variable in position in the popliteal fossa. The superficial varices are marked with a skin marker (Figure 5.3.16).

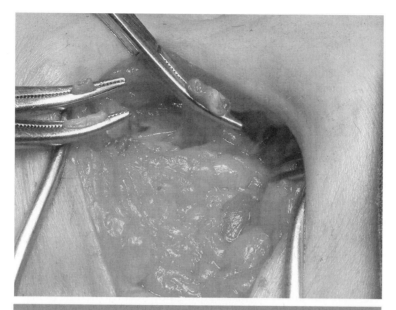

Fig. 5.3.17: The sapheno-popliteal junction has been disconnected and is about to be ligated.

A transverse 4 cm incision is made over the pre-marked site, in the popliteal fossa, over the sapheno-popliteal junction.

A further transverse incision is made in the deep fascia and dissection is carried down, deep to the fascia, to expose the junction between the short saphenous vein and the popliteal vein.

All the tributaries draining into the saphenous vein are ligated and divided. The short saphenous vein is then ligated at its junction with the popliteal vein and divided (Figure 5.3.17).

Stripping of short saphenous vein may be performed, although many surgeons prefer not to do that as it may result in damage to the sural nerve.

Operation for perforators

Sub-fascial endoscopic perforator surgery is used for ligation of incompetent perforators in the case of leg ulcers or to treat lipodermatosclerosis. However, the exact role of this procedure remains controversial.

Complications

The complications are as follows:

1. Bruising and discomfort in the leg.

2. Damage to the sensory nerves, i.e. saphenous or sural nerves.
3. Damage to motor nerves, i.e. femoral in the inguinal region and branches of sciatic in the popliteal fossa.
4. Venous thrombosis in the residual superficial veins.
5. Deep venous thrombosis and incompetence.
6. Recurrence in the long term.

AMPUTATIONS

Indications
Amputation is considered when part of the limb is dead, deadly or a dead loss. The cause may be arterial, venous, neurological or musculoskeletal. However, in modern practice >80% of amputations are due to peripheral vascular disease. These indications include the following two types:

- Vascular
  - Arterial occlusion or stenosis causing non-reconstructible ischaemia.
  - Extensive spreading infection related to moist gangrene.
  - Severe rest pain without gangrene to improve quality of life.
  - Extensive trauma that precludes repair.
- Non-vascular
  - Tumour of bone, soft tissue, muscle, blood vessels and nerves.
  - Severe contractures or paralysis which hinders normal movements.

Assessment
The patient undergoing amputation requires both general assessment as well as assessment to decide the level of amputation.

General assessment
This includes:

- Patient's general condition.
- Feasibility for rehabilitation.

Level of amputation
This depends upon:

- The reason for which it is being considered.
- The status of limb circulation.
- The level of viable tissue;
- Assessment of proximal joints for mobility and contractures.
- The length of stump sufficient for function of prosthesis.

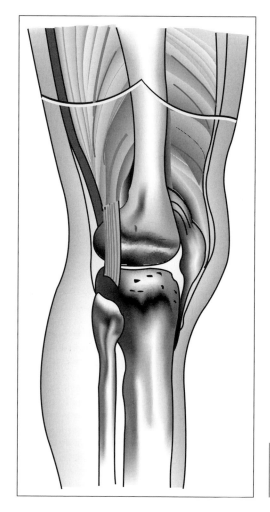

Fig. 5.3.18: Fish-mouth incision for above knee amputation.

Operative technique
Above-knee amputation

Fish-mouth incision (curved equal anterior and posterior skin flaps) is made approximately one and a half times the antero-posterior diameter of the thigh. Skin, deep fascia and muscles are transected at the level of skin incision. Alternatively flaps can be cut to either side (Figures 5.3.18 and 5.3.19).

The vessels are ligated individually and transected.

The sciatic nerve is dissected out. Its accompanying artery is ligated and the nerve pulled down to transect as high as possible.

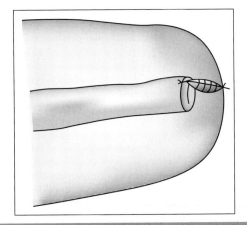

Fig. 5.3.19: A completed above knee amputation.

After retracting muscles and skin the femur is divided well proximal to the soft tissue resection. The end of bone is beveled and haemostasis secured.

The anterior and posterior muscles, and fascia are then stitched together. Suction drain may be placed deep to the muscles. Subcutaneous stitches are used to reduce tension on skin stitches. Skin is closed with interrupted stitches. Transparent dressing is used over the wound, covered by gauze and crepe bandage.

Below-knee amputation
Two types of flaps can be used for below-knee amputation:

1. Long posterior flap.
2. Skew flaps.

The total length of flap/flaps needs to be approximately more than one and a half times the diameter of leg at the point of bone section. For long posterior flap, the anterior skin and soft tissue are cut perpendicular to the long axis of the leg for half the circumference. From there the incision is extended distally to create a long posterior flap.

The bulk of muscles from posterior compartment of leg is left attached to the posterior flap.

Blood vessels are identified and individually ligated and transected. Nerves are pulled down and transected as high as possible after ligating their accompanying vessels.

Periosteum is elevated over both the bones and skin, and muscles are retracted. Fibula is divided 2 cm proximal to the level of tibial division. Tibia is then

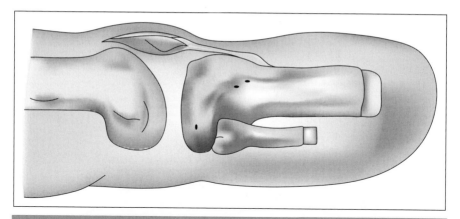

Fig. 5.3.20: In below knee amputation the fibula is divided about 2 cm proximal to the level of the tibia.

cleared and divided obliquely at the appropriate level. The anterior end is then filed and beveled to prevent pressure necrosis of the flap (Figure 5.3.20).

The area is washed, and the muscle and fascia are then sutured anteriorly to bring the flap over the bone. The bulky long posterior flap covers the bone. Suction drain may be placed deep to the muscle. Subcutaneous stitches are used to reduce tension on skin stitches. The skin is closed with interrupted stitches and dressings are applied.

Transmetatarsal (forefoot) amputation

This is done for necrosis or ischaemia involving several toes or the forefoot.

Incision is made with a short dorsal flap, directly over the line of bone trans-action, and a long plantar flap. This is deepened to the bone (Figures 5.3.21 and 5.3.22).

The metatarsals are divided proximal to the level of dorsal incision after dividing the muscles tendons and ligaments. Haemostasis is secured.

The plantar flap is sutured with the dorsal flap to cover the bone ends. Suction drain may be placed deep to the muscle. Subcutaneous stitches are used to reduce tension on skin stitches. Skin is closed with interrupted stitches.

Toe amputation

Amputation of one or more toes may be required for gangrene or osteomyelitis.

A transphalangeal amputation is used if necrosis is distant to the proximal interphalangeal joint without any cellulitis. For more proximal amputation of

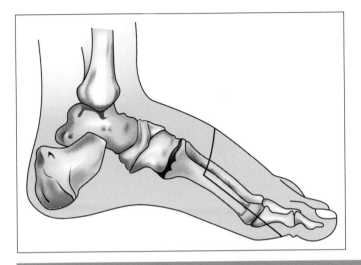

Fig. 5.3.21: The incision for forefoot amputation is made with a long posterior flap.

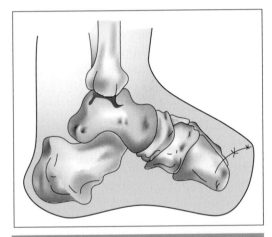

Fig. 5.3.22: A completed forefoot amputation.

a toe, ray amputation is done. This involves the removal of metatarsal head (Figure 5.3.23).

Complications

The complications are follows:

1. Infection.
2. Wound dehiscence.

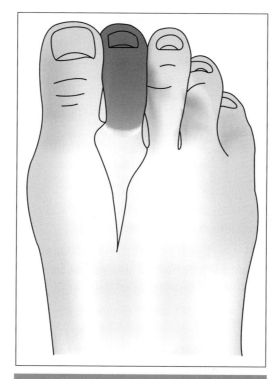

Fig. 5.3.23: Ray amputation for a gangrenous toe.

3. Gangrene of flaps.
4. Phantom pain.
5. Contracture of proximal joint.
6. Chronic pain due to neuroma.
7. Pressure ulcer of stump due to prosthesis.

OPERATIVE TECHNIQUES FOR VASCULAR EMERGENCIES

Embolectomy

This is the procedure to remove fresh embolus or a propagating thrombus, lodged in a vessel obstructing distal blood supply and threatening limb survival. It can be done under general or local anaesthesia.

Femoral embolectomy

Femoral embolectomy is done by making a transverse or vertical incision in the groin and exposing the vessel.

After obtaining proximal and distal control, a transverse or longitudinal arteriotomy is made in common femoral artery.

If the clot is present at that level it extrudes out and is removed. Then a Fogarty catheter of appropriate size is passed proximally and distally. This will remove proximal thrombus from external iliac and common iliac arteries, and distal thrombus from superficial femoral, popliteal and profunda femoris arteries.

Arteries distal to trifurcation of popliteal artery may need to be accessed by an incision below-knee joint if required.

The catheter is passed and then pulled out of the vessel slowly after inflating the balloon. This brings the thrombus/clot out. The procedure is repeated until back bleeding occurs. Inflow from proximal and backflow from distal vessels assesses the effectiveness of embolectomy.

The arteriotomy is then closed with a 5/0 prolene suture. Transverse arteriotomy is closed by simple interrupted stitches but longitudinal arteriotomy requires a vein or prosthetic patch to avoid narrowing at that level.

Brachial embolectomy
Brachial embolectomy is done usually by making a transverse incision in cubital fossa and exposing the brachial artery (Figure 5.3.24).

After obtaining proximal and distal control, a transverse or longitudinal arteriotomy is made. If the clot is present at that level it extrudes out and is removed.

Then a Fogarty catheter of appropriate size is passed proximally and distally. This will remove proximal thrombus from brachial and axillary arteries, and distal thrombus from radial and ulnar arteries (Figures 5.3.25 and 5.3.26).

The arteriotomy is closed with 6/0 prolene. In the case of a longitudinal arteriotomy a vein patch may be required to avoid narrowing the artery.

REPAIR OF RUPTURED AORTIC ANEURYSMS

See repair of abdominal aortic aneurysms.

VASCULAR TRAUMA

Major vascular injuries can be triaged into three main groups:

1. Life-threatening injuries requiring immediate operation.
2. Obvious, stable vascular injuries which can be investigated (arteriogram).
3. Injuries requiring evaluation because of their proximity to vascular structures.

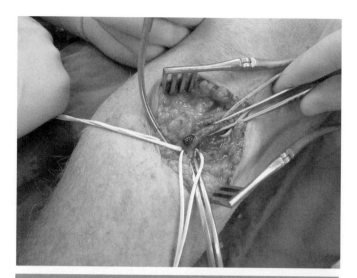

Fig. 5.3.24: Brachial embolectomy. An arteriotomy incision has been made in the brachial artery above its bifurcation with the embolus protruding through the incision.

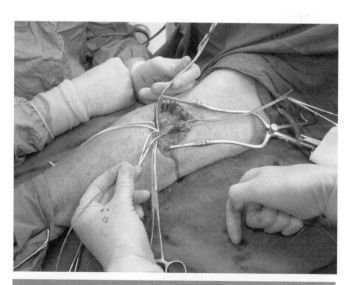

Fig. 5.3.25: A Fogarty balloon catheter is about to be passed into the brachial artery.

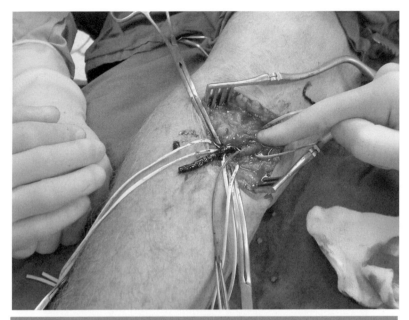

Fig. 5.3.26: The embolus has been removed by pulling out the balloon catheter.

Signs of arterial injury:

1. Expanding or pulsating haematoma.
2. Pulsatile bleeding.
3. Bruit or thrill.
4. End-organ ischaemia.

Signs which may suggest an arterial injury include presence of a stable haematoma, unexplained shock, injury to adjacent nerve or injury in a location likely to involve vascular structure. Distal pulses may still be palpable in the presence of an arterial injury.

Arteriogram is the investigation of choice giving anatomical details of the injury. It should be obtained wherever possible.

Initial management begins with control of haemorrhage. Direct digital pressure is applied at or proximal to the source of bleeding for temporary control. Tourniquets should be avoided because they can cause more tissue damage by blocking all the distal blood supply. Blindly putting haemostats in the wound and removing any debris or embedded material should be avoided.

Operative intervention is timed according to the severity of injury. Patient is prepared thinking that the need to take saphenous vein from leg or to obtain control in the chest may be required. Adequate amount of blood for transfusion with rapid transfusion device should be available.

Proximal and distal arterial control is obtained before approaching the injury. Peri-operative thrombectomy or embolectomy may be required and can be done with a Fogarty catheter. The injured part of the vessel is debrided widely, without compromise considering the mechanism of injury, to ensure a proper repair.

The options for repair include:

1. Simple arteriorraphy.
2. Venous patch angioplasty.
3. Resection of damaged part and end-to-end anastomosis.
4. Interposition graft using saphenous vein.
5. Use of prosthetic grafts is controversial because of the risk of infection.

5.4   THE ROLE OF THE VASCULAR SCRUB NURSE

J. Bell

The peri-operative period consists of three phases: the immediate pre-operative phase including the induction of anaesthesia; the intra-operative phase, beginning from the time the patient is transferred onto the operating table until the time the patient is admitted into recovery and the post-operative period, beginning with the admission of the patient to recovery and ending when the surgeon discontinues follow-up care (*Association of Operating Room Nurses*, 1985; Atkinson, 1992).

PERI-OPERATIVE NURSING

The concept of peri-operative nursing was developed in the 1980s (Mardell, 1998). Peri-operative nurses view the patients holistically and as individuals. Their role is to act as the patients advocate, providing high-quality care throughout all stages of the patients visit to the operating theatre until they are independent of such assistance. Chitwood and Swain (1992) define peri-operative nursing as "providing care for the patient during a period of enforced dependency".

A good peri-operative nurse is one who is well organised, well prepared, and one who remains cool and calm, who has everything to hand and knows where everything is. They are knowledgeable, enthusiastic, motivated and committed to working as part of a multi-disciplinary team, using evidence-based practice and reflection. Peri-operative nurses are actively involved in patient care. They are independent, autonomous practitioners ensuring a strong nursing presence and remains in theatre to protect the needs of the patient. Patients are their main priority.

Peri-operative nurses are busy developing, assessing and planning the patient's surgical care long before the patient enters the operating room to ensure a positive outcome. It is the right of every patient to receive the high-est quality of care according to identified, individual needs.

The peri-operative nurse must provide direct or indirect patient care in a safe environment using nursing judgement, interpersonal skills, communication skills and critical thinking skills.

The peri-operative nurse is a vital member of the surgical team providing necessary support to both the surgeon and anaesthetist as they aim to achieve their ultimate goal, which is providing high-quality patient care.

As a peri-operative nurse, two roles to consider are those of a scrub nurse and of a circulating nurse.

Responsibilities of the vascular scrub nurse

The surgical team consists of the surgeon, surgical assistant, anaesthetist, anaesthetic nurse, scrub person and circulating person. Teamwork by all these personnel is essential to ensure the efficient running of the theatre.

A vascular scrub nurse is a vital member of the vascular surgical team. The vascular scrub nurse possesses skills, knowledge and judgements to help make patient care in the operating room safe, efficient, cost effective and of the highest possible quality.

The scrub nurses major role is to work directly with the surgeon, usually standing directly opposite within the sterile field, passing appropriate instruments, swabs and sutures in a firm manner in the direction of use during the procedure. The surgeon should not have to readjust the instrument once in his hand.

The scrub nurse creates and maintains a sterile field, monitors it constantly to prevent contamination, watches the surgeon constantly, listening and trying to anticipate his needs as the surgery progresses.

The scrub nurse demonstrates workplace safety by following all local policies, procedures, standards, manufactures' guideline, infection control policies, risk management, health and safety, moving and handling and Control Of Substances Hazardous to Health (COSHH) regulations.

Duties before the operation
Duties before the operation include:

- All persons entering the theatre complex should be dressed in surgical attire and footwear wearing hats and masks as per local policy.
- Check theatre is clean, dust free and the operating list is displayed.
- Check surgeon's preference cards and collect specific equipment, sutures and trays of instruments relevant for the procedure.

Vascular instrumentation
- Vascular instrumentation includes clamps which vary in size, curved or double curved, atraumatic to hold vessels firm on the adventitia of the vessel

without causing damage to the intimal layer. They may be fully or partially occlusive, such as the Debakey clamp. This clamp is ring handled with a ratchet lock for partial occlusion allowing work to be carried out on the vessel whilst blood still flows through the remainder.

- Other necessary instruments include retractors, tissue forceps, scissors, haemostatic forceps and sharps.
- Vascular instruments should be sharp and fine in nature to allow for precise work.
- Grafts which may be either straight or bifurcated.
- Embolectomy catheters of various sizes.
- Magnifying loops or glasses.
- Sutures are of the round-bodied type, e.g. Prolene.
- May need X-ray equipment.

Gown and glove to help reduce the risk of infection, using aseptic technique, checking the integrity of the gowns and gloves.

Drape and prepare trolleys with pre-packed instrument trays checking packaging, expiry dates and seals.

Check content of each tray with enclosed list to ensure everything is there.

Collect all necessary "extras" for the case.

Count swabs, needles and instruments with the circulating nurse prior to commencement of the operation as per local policy.

Check patient details are correct, including consent, allergies, and limb marking with the notes and circulating nurse.

Ensure the patient is safely positioned on the operating table.

Duties during the operation
Duties during the operation include the following:

- Create the sterile field as close as possible to the time of use, the patient being at the centre, maintaining integrity, safety and efficiency of the sterile field throughout the procedure. If sterility is in doubt, consider it unsterile.
- Prepare and hand skin preparation sponges to the surgeon.
- Assist in draping.
- Position trolleys to create a sterile field.
- Connect suction, diathermy, checking settings with the surgeon.
- Prepare the work area.
- Use sterile items within the sterile field.
- Pass instruments in an efficient manner using a hands-free method with sharp instruments.

- Keep an accurate swab, needle and instrument count throughout.
- Anticipate the needs of the surgeon by continually observing the progress of the operation.
- Before closing any orifice a count must be performed and the surgeon informed of the findings. Ensure the surgeon acknowledges the information. If there is an incorrect count local policies must be followed.

Duties at the end of the operation

Duties at the end of the operation include the following:

- Ensure correct dressing is applied.
- Final checks performed of swabs, needles and instruments.
- Drapes removed to ensure patient is clean and the wound dry, and any drains unclamped.
- Cover the patient to ensure dignity and warmth.
- De-gown and de-glove, clear away instruments and sharps as per local policy.
- Complete all relevant documentation. Patient care must be documented on pre-printed care plans, individualised to patients needs, so that the care provided is evident and not kept as a secret. This will help validate peri-operative nursing practices and provide direction for the education of peri-operative nurses (Parker & Cheryl, 1999).

Responsibilities of the circulating nurse (runner)

The circulating nurse is another vital member of the surgical team providing for the safety and comfort of the surgical patient outside the sterile field.

Duties before operation

Their role before the operation includes:

- Acting as the unsterile member of the team.
- Ensuring the operating room is clean and fully stocked.
- Checking all equipment is present and in working order.
- Ensuring temperature and humidity are correct.
- Opening sterile trays and packs.
- Assisting with the count and recording it in the relevant documents.
- Pouring solutions carefully to avoid splashing.

Duties during operation

During the operation the circulating nurse's role includes:

- Remaining in theatre throughout the operation.
- Connecting necessary equipment.

- Replenish and record swabs, packs and needles as required.
- Adhere to local policy on disposal of swabs.
- Ensure theatre doors remain closed and traffic is kept to a minimum.
- Anticipate needs of the surgical team.
- Constantly monitor and maintain the sterile field.
- Labels any specimens correctly with the appropriate form.

Duties before the end of operation

Duties before the end of the operation include:

- Assist with counts and documentation.
- Prepare wound dressings.

Duties on completion of the operation

Duties on completion of the operation include:

- Tidy up, removing drapes and dirty instruments as per local policy.
- Help remove the patient safely to recovery.
- Ensure the operating room is cleaned and prepared for the next case.

Both the scrub nurse and circulating nurse play a vital role as members of the vascular surgical team. If the desired outcome of safe, effective, high-quality patient care is to be achieved then teamwork by all personnel is a necessity.

REFERENCES

Association of Operating Room Nurses (1985) A model for peri-operative nursing practice. *Assoc Operat Room Nurse J* 41: 188–193.

Atkinson LJ (1992) *Berry & Kohn's Operating Room Technique,* 7th Edition. St. Louis, London, Mosby.

Chitwood LB (1992) *Peri-operative Nursing: A Study and Learning Tool.* Springhouse Corporation, Pennsylvania.

Clarke P & Jones J (1998) *Brigden's Operating Department Practice.* Churchill Livingstone, Edinburgh.

Mardell A (1998) How theatre nurses perceive their role: a study. *Nurs Stand* 13(9): 45–47.

McGarvey HE (2000) Development and definition of the role of the operating department nurse: a review. *J Adv Nurs* 32(5): 1092–1100.

Parker & Cheryl B (1999) Clinical decision – making processes in peri-operative nursing. *Assoc Operat Room Nurse J* 70(1): 45–46, 48, 50, 52, 56, 58, 61–62.

Scott E, Earl C, Leaper D & Massey M (1999) Understanding peri-operative nursing. *Nurs Stand* 13(49): 49–54.

West, Bernice JM (1992) *Theatre Nursing. Technique and Care,* 6th Edition. Baillière Tindall, London.

SUGGESTED FURTHER READING

Bellman L & Manley K (2000) *Surgical Nursing: Advancing Practice.* Churchill Livingstone.

Murray S (2001) *Vascular Disease – Nursing and Management.* Whurr Publishers. ISBN 1861562195.

Nightingale K (1999) *Understanding Peri-operative Nursing.* JW Arrowsmith Limited. Arnold.

Phippen ML & Wells MP (2000) *Patient Care during Operative and Invasive Procedures.* WB Saunders Company.

5.5 POST-OPERATIVE CARE OF VASCULAR SURGERY PATIENTS

J.C. Watts

INTRODUCTION

Crucial to ensuring good outcomes for surgical patients is returning them from theatre to an environment where they can receive the correct level of care, and to pay appropriate attention to the detail of that care.

"Levels of care" have been redefined by the Department of Health (DoH) ("Comprehensive Critical Care" DoH, 2000) and are detailed in Table 5.5.1.

Depending upon circumstances, the needs of some patients may be adequately met on an "ordinary" ward, whilst others may require admission to a specialist treatment area, such as an intensive care or high-dependency unit. For clarity, the term "critical care unit" (CCU) will be used as a generic term for these areas in this chapter.

LEVELS OF CARE

Whilst unexpected complications can always arise during surgery and anaesthesia, the decision about where a patient should be nursed after their operation should be made before surgery occurs depending upon the level of care it is anticipated that they will require.

Many patients can be returned to an "ordinary" ward rather than a CCU if the environment is appropriate.

If the patient requires a particular type of post-operative intervention which is not available on an "ordinary" ward (e.g. cardiac monitoring, advanced pain relieving techniques, etc.), then they should be nursed in an environment that has the appropriate facilities. In some hospitals this may only be available in the CCU, but in others there may be more appropriate environments available. If these facilities are not available on the day of surgery, this may mean cancellation of the operation.

Table 5.5.1: Definition of "levels of care" (from "comprehensive critical care" DoH, 2000)

Level	Description	Example
0	Patients whose needs can be met through normal ward care in an acute hospital	Day-case patient, or patient undergoing "minor surgery" requiring in patient stay. Patients requiring standard monitoring and standard interventions
1	Patients at risk of their condition deteriorating, or those recently relocated from higher levels of care, whose needs can be met on an acute ward with additional advice and support from the critical care team	Traditional "monitored bed", e.g. isolated (but stable) cardiac problem. Patients with a stable co-existing medical disease, or who have undergone medium/major surgery without complication
2	Patients requiring more detailed observation or intervention including support for a single failing organ system or post-operative care and those stepping down from higher levels of care	Traditional "high-dependency unit", e.g. cardiac and respiratory problems, advanced pain relief techniques, coronary care, etc. Patients with severe medical diseases, or those who have undergone major surgery, and who are at risk of complications
3	Patients requiring advanced respiratory support alone; or basic respiratory support together with support of at least two organ systems. This level includes all complex patients requiring support for multi-organ failure	Traditional "intensive care", e.g. respiratory failure, sepsis, etc. Patients with severe life-threatening illness, trauma, some forms of major surgery, etc.

POST-OPERATIVE RECOVERY

Immediately after the anaesthetic

After surgery, the patient enters what is termed as the "recovery period". In most cases following a general anaesthetic (GA), the anaesthetic is turned off, and the patient will begin to breathe independently of the ventilator. When the patient is breathing on their own, they will be removed from the ventilator and allowed to go to the "recovery room", breathing oxygen.

In the recovery room, the patient receives "one-to-one nursing". Physiological parameters are measured and recorded. If the patient remains stable, they will

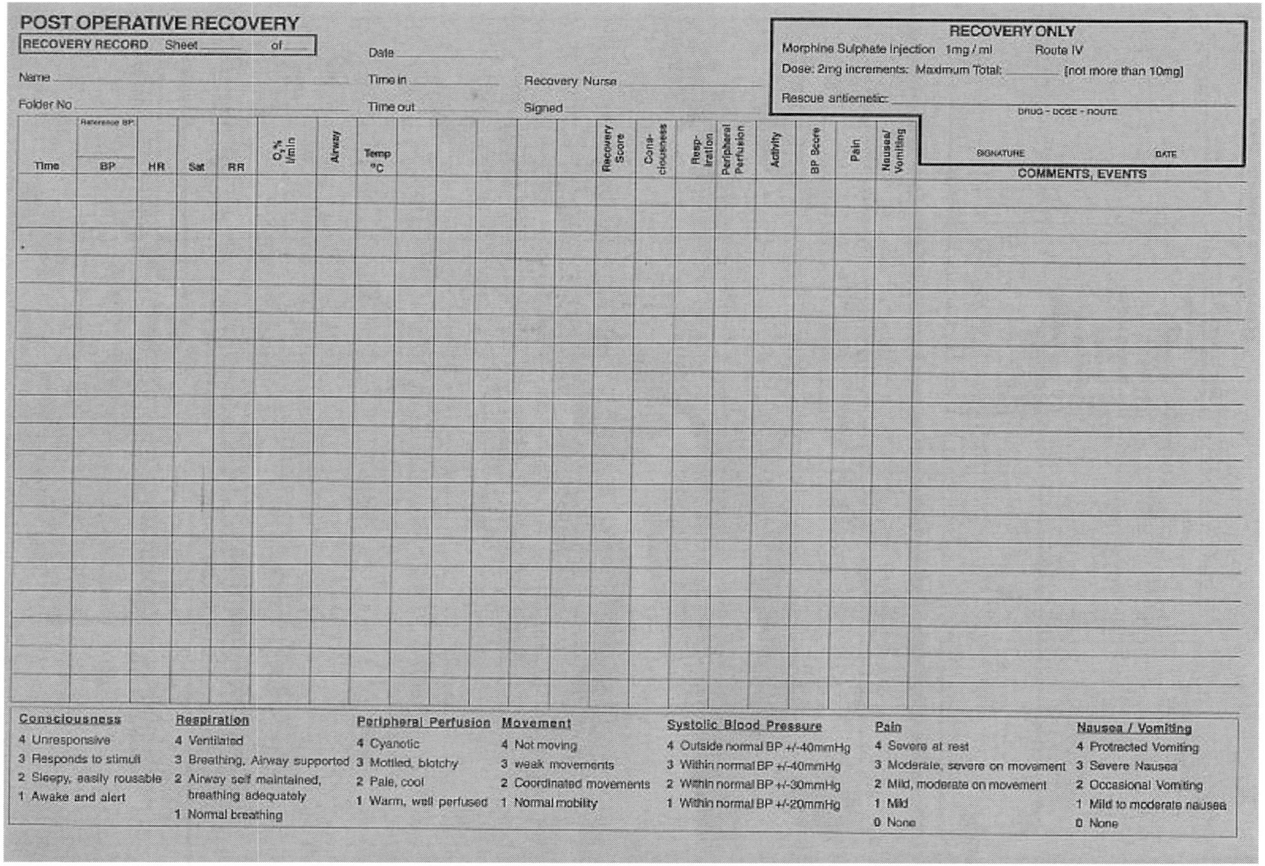

POST OPERATIVE RECOVERY

RECOVERY RECORD Sheet ______ of ______

Date ______

Name ______ Time in ______ Recovery Nurse ______

Folder No ______ Time out ______ Signed ______

RECOVERY ONLY

Morphine Sulphate Injection 1mg / ml Route IV

Dose: 2mg increments: Maximum Total: ______ [not more than 10mg]

Rescue antiemetic: ______ DRUG - DOSE - ROUTE

SIGNATURE DATE

Time	Reference BP: BP	HR	Sat	RR	O_2% l/min	Airway	Temp °C						Recovery Score	Cons-ciousness	Resp-iration	Peripheral Perfusion	Activity	BP Score	Pain	Nausea/ Vomiting	COMMENTS, EVENTS

Consciousness
4 Unresponsive
3 Responds to stimuli
2 Sleepy, easily rousable
1 Awake and alert

Respiration
4 Ventilated
3 Breathing, Airway supported
2 Airway self maintained, breathing adequately
1 Normal breathing

Peripheral Perfusion
4 Cyanotic
3 Mottled, blotchy
2 Pale, cool
1 Warm, well perfused

Movement
4 Not moving
3 weak movements
2 Coordinated movements
1 Normal mobility

Systolic Blood Pressure
4 Outside normal BP +/-40mmHg
3 Within normal BP +/-40mmHg
2 Within normal BP +/-30mmHg
1 Within normal BP +/-20mmHg

Pain
4 Severe at rest
3 Moderate, severe on movement
2 Mild, moderate on movement
1 Mild
0 None

Nausea / Vomiting
4 Protracted Vomiting
3 Severe Nausea
2 Occasional Vomiting
1 Mild to moderate nausea
0 None

Fig. 5.5.1: A typical recovery room chart.

be discharged from the recovery area to the ward which will care for them. Recovery rooms need the facilities to care for patients for prolonged periods of time if need be.

Patients who have undergone elective surgery will often be recovered in this way if they have had a straightforward operation without complicating medical or surgical factors. On occasions, they may remain on a ventilator for some hours, and be transferred in that manner to the CCU. Emergency vascular patients will commonly remain ventilated for some time after the procedure (Figure 5.5.1).

Critical care units (Level 2 and Level 3 care)

CCUs have a larger nursing/patient ratio than "ordinary" wards. Critical care nursing is a challenging combination of thorough basic nursing care and technology. However, the most important factors are attention to detail, and a well-founded understanding of when and why interventions are required.

Basic nursing considerations

Table 5.5.2 illustrates the main issues surrounding basic nursing care in vascular patients. Post-operative patients may be fully conscious and able to express their needs and requirements. However, they may also be confused, in a coma, or under sedation.

Figure 5.5.2 shows a standard post-operative observation chart.

The minimum post-operative observations for *all* post-operative surgical patients are:

- *Respiratory rate*: An abnormal respiratory rate is often the first indication that the patient is deteriorating. Abnormal respiratory rates on admission to CCU are an independent indicator of poor outcome in critically ill patients.
- *Pulse rate*: The significance of the pulse rate will depend partially upon the patient's normal resting pulse rate. Fast, slow and irregular pulses can all have serious complications.
- *Blood pressure*: This is an indication of how well the heart is pumping blood around the body. If blood pressure is adequate, then the body's organs will be properly perfused with oxygen. If the organs are not properly perfused, they will eventually fail.
- *Peripheral pulses and limb monitoring*: Cool or discoloured limbs, and poor pulses can indicate ischaemia, requiring urgent surgical intervention.
- *Conscious level*: This can be assessed using the Glasgow Coma Scale (GCS), which measures the patient's response to various stimuli. This is scored out

Table 5.5.2: Basic nursing care issues in the vascular patient

Area of care	Nursing issues
Skin care	• Pressure area care • Cannulae sites
Nutrition	• Dietry requirements • Assistance with feeding • Parenteral feeding • Blood-sugar measurement in diabetic patients
Hygiene	• Toiletry needs • Catheter care • Oral hygiene • Tracheostomy care • Infection control issues
Basic observations	• Respiratory rate • Pulse rate • Blood pressure • Urine output • Conscious level • Temperature
Vascular surgery specific observations	• Peripheral pulses • Limb colour • Limb temperature
Comfort	• Pain relief from operation • Other causes of discomfort
Dignity	• Privacy and respect • Visitors • Confidentiality • Communication

of 15 possible points, where 15/15 is equivalent to "alert and orientated", and 8/15 is generally equivalent to "coma". A score of 3/15 means that the patient is totally unresponsive. However, it is important to remember that interpretation of the score is subject to context: a score of 3/15 will not distinguish a patient who is dead on arrival in hospital from one who is anaesthetised!

However, conscious level can be quickly assessed using the alert, verbal, painful, unresponsive (AVPU) scale (Table 5.5.3).

It is also important to observe whether the patient is orientated in time and space (whether they remember where they are, and what the date and time is) as disorientation can herald the onset of confusion.

The Early Warning Scoring System

All patients should be scored on admission and then once daily.
Patients requiring frequent observations are to be scored each time.
To be used at any time on any patient who may be at risk of their condition deteriorating.
Once scored please use the flow chart for further action.

SCORE	3	2	1	0	1	2	3
Response to stimulus				Alert	Voice	Pain	Unresp.
Temp.		>35°C		35°C–37.5°C	>37.6–38.4°C	>38.5°C	
Systolic BP	Normal systolic BP – 50mmHg	Normal systolic BP – 30-40mmHg	Normal Systolic BP – 20mmHg	Patient's Normal systolic BP	Normal systolic BP + 20mm Hg	Normal systolic BP + 30-40mmHg	Normal systolic BP + 50mmHg
Heart Rate		<40	40–50	51–100	101–110	111–129	>130
Respiratory Rate		<8		9–14	15–20	21–29	>30
Urine output	Nil	<30 mls/hr	<50 mls/hr		>100 mls/hr		

This scoring system has been adapted for Burnley General Hospital from the Modified Early Warning Scoring System used at Queens Hospital Burton-Upon-Trent, first devised at James Paget Hospital, Great Yarmouth.
Critical Care Outreach Sister Julie Sharpley [May 2002]

SURGICAL FLOW CHART

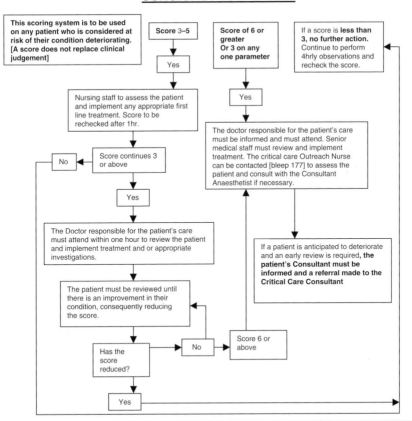

Fig. 5.5.2: Burnley EW chart from a surgical ward.

Table 5.5.3: The AVPU scale

	Definition	Approximate GCS equivalent
A	Patient is **A**lert and orientated	15/15
V	Patient responds to **V**erbal cues	13/15
P	Patient responds to **P**ainful stimuli	10/15
U	Patient is **U**nresponsive	<8/15

Differences in movements between the left and right side of the body may indicate a stroke, and should also be recorded.

- *Temperature*: High temperatures may herald post-operative infection. Hypothermia can be caused by prolonged operations, or by impaired patient metabolism. Both can be serious, and should be treated appropriately.

OTHER CONSIDERATIONS

Patients who require respiratory support

"Respiratory support" ranges from supplementary oxygen therapy to full mechanical ventilation. Oxygen therapy must be controlled and prescribed properly. Table 5.5.4 illustrates the different types of support available, although not all hospitals can supply all types.

"Mechanical ventilation" is the use of an external mechanical device to assist or take over the breathing of a patient. This can involve ventilation through a tight-fitting face mask (non-invasive positive pressure ventilation – NIPPV), or ventilation via an endotracheal tube (a tube into the windpipe: invasive positive pressure ventilation – IPPV). Ventilators use "positive pressure", driving oxygen "under force" into the lungs.

Mechanical ventilation initially requires that the patient is heavily sedated and can predispose to chest infections and respiratory problems if prolonged. It is therefore important to anticipate, detect and treat respiratory difficulties early to prevent the patient being mechanically ventilated, and to keep periods of ventilation as short as possible. The process of removing someone from mechanical ventilation is called "weaning".

When being ventilated, the functioning of the ventilator – including how much oxygen is being delivered – will need to be monitored, as well as additional patient parameters, such as oxygen saturation, and expired carbon dioxide levels.

Table 5.5.4: Different types of respiratory support

Type of respiratory support	Equipment	Function mode	Description	Type of patient
Oxygen therapy via mask/nasal cannulae	• Face mask (various types) • Nasal cannulae	Patient's own respiratory drive	Normal air contains 21% oxygen. Many patients will require a higher concentration post-operatively even for a short period	All patients, although caution in some with chronic lung disease
Continuous positive airway pressure (CPAP)	• Tight-fitting mask • Supplemental oxygen • CPAP valve device	Patient's own respiratory drive	Prevents collapse of small areas of lung, improving oxygen transfer into the blood	Patients with chronic chest problems or severe chest infections
NIPPV	• Tight-fitting facemask • Mechanical ventilator • Oxygen supply	External ventilator and/or patient's own respiratory drive	A ventilator assists the patient to breathe via a tight-fitting face mask. Techniques employed range from assistance to full ventilation	Patients with chronic chest problems can prevent progression to IPPV
IPPV	• Mechanical ventilator • Endotracheal tube • Oxygen supply	Full mechanical ventilation through a tube in the windpipe	A ventilator assists the patient to breathe via an endotracheal tube. Sedation is often required	Patients with respiratory failure or undergoing anaesthesia

Patients who require cardiovascular support

Blood pressure needs to be maintained to ensure that all organs have an adequate supply of oxygen. A low blood pressure can be caused by several clinical problems (see Table 5.5.5).

The left side of the heart is a pump which pushes oxygenated blood around the body. Anything which impairs the pumping strength of the heart muscle (e.g. heart failure, fluid overload, fluid under load, dysrythmia, etc.) can result in "left-sided heart failure", with low blood pressure, poor urine output and

Table 5.5.5: Causes of low blood pressure

	Non-cardiac causes	Cardiac causes
Description	Loss of circulating volume (e.g. haemorrhage) Dehydration from excessive fluid losses	Cardiac failure (fluid overload, heart attack, "poor pumping", dysrhythmia, etc.)
Treatment	Fluid replacement therapy Blood transfusion	Treat causes (e.g. diuretics) Treat cardiac dysrhythmias (e.g. digoxin) Improve heart pumping (e.g. inotropic medication) Administration of nitrates

pulmonary oedema. Treatment includes resuscitative measures, administration of oxygen and diuretics. Dysrhythmias may require specific drug treatment. However, if these treatments are not effective, the patient may also require inotropic drugs which support the blood pressure. These are given as continuous infusions. There are several types of inotropic drugs, each with differing actions. The exact drug prescribed will depend upon clinical circumstances.

Patients who are at risk of sudden deterioration

Deterioration can be "anticipated" (due to the nature of a pre-existing condition or the type of surgery undergone) or unanticipated. It is important to remember that unanticipated deteriorations can be due to equipment failure, or idiosyncratic reactions to therapy (e.g. drug allergy) as well as unexpected conditions, such as heart attack, or pulmonary embolus. Proper attention to basic patient care and monitoring can prevent or allow early detection of some of these conditions.

Monitoring

Patients are often taken to CCU for "monitoring". Primarily, this will be for observation of basic physiological data as described above. The importance of meticulous fluid balance recording as part of this process cannot be overemphasised.

A variety of additional monitors can be utilised depending upon the patient's clinical need. These are detailed in Table 5.5.6.

Monitors alone do not guarantee the safety of the patient. It is a correct interpretation of the data supplied by the monitors that is important. It is vital that staff using the monitors understand how they work, how to calibrate them

Table 5.5.6: Monitors commonly used on CCU

Monitor	Explanation	Notes
Pulse oximetry	A monitor can be attached to the nose, ear or digit. Absorption of infrared light by the tissue is measured. The saturation of blood with oxygen is displayed as a percentage. Values of <94% may indicate impending hypoxia. Additionally, the device can measure pulse rate and rhythm	• Abnormal blood pigments may cause inaccuracy • Pressure from the probe may cause tissue necrosis
ECG	Measures heart electrical activity. Heart rate and rhythm are displayed. Signs of impending cardiac ischaemia can be detected	• Movement and electrical apparatus cause inaccuracy
Capnography	A monitor inserted into the breathing tubes which can detect carbon dioxide.	• Indicates that ventilation is occurring
Ventilator monitors	Airway pressure, breath volume and inspired oxygen levels are all monitored	• Demonstrate that ventilator is working correctly • Ensure that correct pressure and oxygen concentrations are being delivered
Syringe drivers and related devices	Rate, driving pressure, power status (e.g. battery low)	• Ensure pumps are working correctly
Central venous pressure (CVP) line	A catheter inserted into a major vein, (usually in the neck) for the administration of drugs, or for the measurement of pressures near the heart CVP. A raised CVP can indicate fluid overload or right heart failure; a low CVP can indicate hypovolaemis	• Can cause cardiac dysrhythmias • Prolonged use may lead to infection • Insertion can cause to other structures
Pulmonary artery flotation catheter (PAFC)	A catheter threaded through major veins, passing through the chambers of the heart, into the pulmonary artery. It can be used to measure the "pumping ability" of the heart (cardiac output) and the pulmonary artery wedge pressure (PAWP)	• As CVP line • Should only be used for a short period of time • Insertion requires more skill than a CVP line
Arterial line	A cannula inserted into an artery (commonly radial) allowing beat-to-beat measurement of blood pressure and repeated blood sampling	• Can cause ischaemia if compromise blood supply • Cannot be used for the administration of drugs

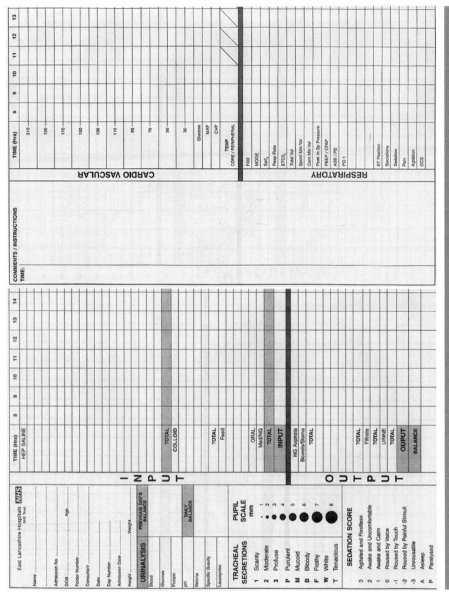

Fig. 5.5.3: A typical CCU observation chart.

and how they can malfunction. Additionally, one set of results from monitors may mean nothing in itself. In the same way that the plot of a film cannot be derived from one still, a set of data from monitors can only be properly interpreted in the context of the trends of the data over the previous few hours. A systolic blood pressure of 90 mmHg may be an alarming finding in isolation; however it may be a reassuring finding if an hour ago before intervention the pressure was 75 mmHg. It is important that after an intervention is performed the patient's condition is re-examined to determine the response to the treatment. All post-operative observation charts should allow this analysis. CCU charts (Figure 5.5.3) allow space for all relevant observations in 24 h to be displayed in relation to therapeutic interventions, allowing response to the intervention to be gauged.

POST-OPERATIVE COMPLICATIONS

These can be classified according to the framework shown in Table 5.5.7.

Co-existing medical disease

The patient must be treated holistically and not just as an interesting surgical problem. Many vascular patients will be elderly and have co-existing medical illnesses that can complicate anaesthesia, surgery and recovery.
Some specific problems are considered below.

Table 5.5.7: Post-operative complications

Type of complication	Examples
Related to co-existing medical disease	• Diabetes • Ischaemic heart disease • Respiratory illness • Arthritis • Age, etc.
General complications related to major surgery	• Post-operative pain • Haemorrhage • Wound infection • Hypothermia • Metabolic disturbances
General complications related to anaesthesia	• Chest complications • Reactions to drugs • Prolonged recovery
Complications related to specific type of vascular surgery undergone	• Emboli/blockages • Stroke • Major haemorrhage

Age

Elderly patients, even if regarded as "fit", will not have the same physiological reserve as younger patients. This means that they will not recover as quickly from illnesses, and are more likely to suffer complications post-operatively. Post-operative confusion is particularly common in those over 80. Age alone should not normally be a bar to admission to a CCU as the decision not to admit should always be based on the assessment as to whether the patient is expected to benefit from invasive treatment and monitoring.

Diabetes

Poor blood sugar control will impair the patient's recovery by promoting infection, and slow wound healing. Most hospitals will have a set guideline devised by the diabetologists to ensure that diabetic surgical patients are cared for appropriately. These will usually involve a post-operative infusion of insulin according to a sliding scale, and an infusion of a set concentration of dextrose, which will be discontinued when the patient is able to return to their normal diabetic regimen. It is important that the patient receives both infusions together: if dextrose only is administered, hyperglycaemia can result; whereas the administration of insulin only will result in hypoglycaemia. These infusions are usually given through a dedicated cannula via infusion pumps, and it is essential that the function and patency of these is checked at regular intervals. Tight blood sugar control has been shown to improve the survival of patients after heart attacks, and those who are critically ill.

Ischaemic heart disease

This is common in vascular surgical patients, and they are at high risk of post-operative cardiac events, such as dysrhythmias and heart attacks. Whilst such events may not be preventable, it is important that the level of risk has been determined pre-operatively so that surgery and anaesthesia can be tailored appropriately.

Strokes

Patients with peripheral vascular disease may also have a degree of carotid artery disease. They may have a history of "transient ischaemic attacks" (mini strokes) or blackouts. They often have a history of high blood pressure, which means that they are often at risk of stroke from hypotension of whatever origin.

Renal function

Vascular patients often have a degree of impaired kidney function, although this may not be symptomatic. Aortic surgery may precipitate post-operative renal failure, particularly if the artery has been clamped for a long time.

Cigarette smoking and lung disease

A history of smoking is associated with more than a three times increase in post-operative lung problems. Even stopping smoking for a short period of time reduces this risk substantially. In the long term, smoking is a major risk factor for global lung diseases, such as asthma and chronic lung disease. Reduced lung function is associated with an increase in post-operative lung problems, and may necessitate post-operative ventilation. In severe lung disease, weaning the patient from mechanical ventilation can be prolonged.

Problems arising from surgery and anaesthesia
Pain relief

Vascular surgery often requires large invasive procedures. Adequate pain relief is important not just on a humanitarian basis, but because it aids the patients recovery, physically and psychologically. If the patient's pain is under control from the moment they are awake, this is better than trying to treat established pain from inadequate analgesia.

Poor post-operative pain relief can impair patient recovery and predispose to complications (e.g. chest infection following inability to cough). All staff should know how to adequately assess a patient's pain. As pain is a subjective experience, it is best to ask the patient! Many methods of assessing pain levels are available, but simple numerical scales (e.g. 0–4 where 0 = "no pain" and 4 = "worst ever pain") are easy to perform and provide results independent of observer bias.

The traditional method of post-operative analgesia of administering opioid drugs (morphine, pethidine, etc.) either regularly, or on patient demand, as intramuscular injections, was inadequate in many ways. Dosages and timings used were often inflexible, pain relief could be uneven, and ward staff were often left to "catch up" on pain relief with unsatisfactory results.

A continuous intravenous infusion of an opioid drug provides better level of analgesia, and can be adjusted to meet the patient's personal requirements. However, there is a risk that the patient could be "accidently overdosed" if the pump malfunctions. Continuous infusions have been replaced in many hospitals by patient-controlled analgesia (PCA) devices. These are essentially pumps containing a solution of opioid (e.g. morphine, 50 mg in 50 ml) which can be adjusted to deliver a set dosage at a set time interval, whenever the patient presses a button (e.g. 1 mg administered every 5 min). A maximum dosage can be set on some devices, which reduces the possibility of overdosage. A PCA places the patient in control of their own pain relief. Studies have shown that the total amount of opioid drug used after operations is lower in patients who use PCAs compared to traditional methods, but their satisfaction with pain relief is higher.

Patients who are prescribed post-operative opioid analgesic drugs should also be prescribed regular anti-emetic medication, as opioids can induce nausea and vomiting. Respiratory depression is the life-threatening side effect, and respiratory rate should be regularly monitored. Overdose is treated with naloxone.

Opioids work best as part of a balanced analgesia regime, utilising regular doses of milder analgesics (e.g. paracetamol) in combination. Typically, if there are no contraindications, a post-operative patient will receive regular paracetamol, a non-steroidal drug (voltarol, feldene, etc.) and opioids, with regular anti-emetic medication. Non-steroidal drugs can reduce the amount of morphine required by a patient, but should be used with caution in patients with a history of stomach ulcers and renal problems.

Regional anaesthesia

Regional anaesthesia (RA) uses local anaesthetic techniques to provide anaesthesia for surgery or pain relief afterwards. Many abdominal procedures will utilise either a spinal or epidural anaesthetic with a GA, as they reduce the total amount of anaesthetic required to keep the patient asleep and comfortable during the operation; also, depending upon the technique used, the effects of the regional anaesthetic can be continued into the post-operative period to provide good analgesia. RA utilises local anaesthetic agents to provide large areas of numbness on the body. It is important that the level of numbness produced by the local anaesthetic is regularly examined, as an excessive block can result in respiratory difficulty and hypotension. If the block is inadequate, pain relief will be poor. Paralysis of the lower body can be a distressing side effect, but resolves when the local anaesthesia wears off. Urinary catheterisation may also be necessary.

An epidural involves placing a catheter into the epidural space which surrounds large nerves as they emerge into the spinal canal from the spinal cord. An epidural can utilise a slow infusion of local anaesthetic (with or without an opioid drug) to provide good quality pain relief post-operatively. If opioids have been used, patients can also suffer from the usual side effects, such as drowsiness and respiratory depression, as well as itchiness. These are usually treated by administering naloxone.

A spinal usually involves a "one shot" injection of local anaesthetic solution into the cerebrospinal fluid (CSF) surrounding the spinal cord. The effects are similar to that of an epidural, but do not usually persist as long.

Prolonged procedure

A major vascular procedure will normally last between 2 and 3 h, but can be prolonged if complications occur. This can result in metabolic disturbances (low sodium and low blood sugar) and hypothermia. Patients may require a period of ventilation in CCU for these abnormalities to be corrected. Pressure areas are also of concern. Patients with vascular disease have poor skin circulation, and are more susceptable to developing pressure sores.

Haemorrhage

Blood loss in most vascular surgery will be small, although the potential for major blood loss is large. In emergency cases, severe haemorrhage may have already occurred before the operation. Blood loss can also occur post-operatively, and may necessitate a return to theatre. It is important that haemoglobin and clotting levels are checked post-operatively.

POST-OPERATIVE PROBLEMS ARISING FROM VASCULAR SURGERY

Renal failure

A degree of pre-existing renal failure is common in vascular patients even if this is not symptomatic. Poor urine output after surgery can be caused by a variety of problems. The kidneys are also sensitive to periods of hypoxia and hypotension.

If there is a low urine output (Table 5.5.8) following surgery, the following strategy is adopted:

1. If the patient is not catheterised, ask about the urge to pass urine, and check if the bladder is distended and palpable. Catheterisation may be required at this point.
2. If the patient is already catheterised, check that it is not displaced or blocked.

Table 5.5.8: Causes of poor urine output

Cause of low urine output	Description	Example
Pre-renal causes	Inadequate kidney perfusion	• Low cardiac output • Low blood pressure • Blood loss
Renal causes	Inadequate kidney function	• Kidney failure (acute/chronic) • Toxic drug effects (e.g. non-steroidal anti-inflammatory drugs (NSAIDs), antibiotics)
Post-renal causes	Inadequate outflow from the kidney	• Blocked catheter • Prostate disease • Regional anaesthetic

3. Check the patient's observations. If they are under hydrated, or hypotensive, the kidneys will not be perfused and intravenous fluid balance should be checked, and fluid prescribed. If the patient is overhydrated, a diuretic may be required to promote urine production.
4. If the cause of low urine output is poor heart function, then the cardiac condition will require to be optimised. This may mean moving the patient to a higher level of care.

During the surgery, the aorta is clamped, and blood flow to the kidney can be impaired. This can be enough for the patient to develop full renal failure. In some cases, this will be reversible with time and renal support therapy. A small number of patients will develop chronic renal failure, and will require long-term dialysis.

Emboli/blockages

The peripheral pulses of post-operative vascular patients must be monitored as part of the routine observations. Blockages in the grafts or vessels are common post-operatively, and may manifest by the loss of a pulse, as well as other signs of poor circulation (skin discolouration, pain, parasthesia, etc.) Signs of poor circulation require an urgent vascular surgery opinion. Ultrasound Doppler is useful in checking flow through the vessels. If a physical vessel blockage, such as an emboli or blood clot is suspected, the patient may be returned to theatre for an urgent revascularisation procedure. Atrial fibrillation is common in elderly patients, and is the usual "default" cardiac rhythm at times of physiological stress. Atrial fibrillation can lead to emboli and strokes or peripheral ischaemia or pulmonary emboli. It is best treated by correcting physiological abnormalities, cardioversion or drugs, such as digoxin or amiodarone. Often these complications occur despite the use of post-operative anticoagulation.

SUPPLEMENTARY AREAS OF CARE

As well as standard nursing issues regarding patient well-being the following should be considered in CCU patients.

Patients who are sedated

Sedation is commenced to allow patients to tolerate the CCU environment and interventions, particularly IPPV. Ideally, the patient will be able to communicate in some form, but sometimes they may be fully anaesthetised. Difficulties can occur when sedation is withdrawn, including anxiety, confusion and withdrawal syndromes.

Prolonged stay in critical care

Most vascular patients will only require 24–48 h in CCU post-operatively. A significant minority of patients may require a longer stay. These are commonly patients with pre-existing concurrent medical illnesses, those who are frail, emergency patients, patients who have had long, complicated procedures or who have developed post-operative complications. These patients are at risk of problems which are associated with a prolonged intensive therapy unit (ITU) stay, such as secondary infection, and may require supplementary surgical procedures (e.g. tracheostomy).

Poor nutrition

Many surveys have found that malnutrition is very common in hospital inpatients. Prolonged periods of illness will worsen this situation, particularly if the patient is "nil by mouth" for a long period of time. Post-operatively, it is important to establish oral (enteral) feeding as soon as possible to protect the gut lining, and complications associated with abdominal problems. This can be established using nasogastric or nasojejunal tubes. In some cases, a feeding port is created directly into the stomach during surgery, or by utilising a percutaneous endoscopic gastrostomy (PEG) technique. Direct access into the small intestine via a jejunostomy is also useful.

In some cases, this is not possible, and the patient will require intravenous feeding. It is important that nutrients, such as vitamins are also administered to prevent deficiency problems. Parenteral feeding is associated with line infections, and colonisation with bacteria.

Muscle weakness

Muscle weakness and subsequent contractures can develop due to prolonged immobility. Additionally, nerve and muscle problems are associated with critical illness ("ITU polyneuropathy", and "ITU polymyopathy"). These alone can lead to a prolonged hospital stay. It is essential that both physiotherapists and occupational therapists are involved appropriately in the care of patients from an early stage. A high awareness of the problem, so that early referral to a rehabilitation facility can be made, is also required.

Psychological disturbances

Symptoms of psychological disturbance have been reported even after short periods of stay in CCU, ranging from amnesia to frank psychosis. A form of post-traumatic stress disorder, incorporating psychotic delusions, based upon "flashbacks" or misinterpreted clinical events, can develop. Access to appropriate counselling can resolve most of these episodes. It is important to remember that the patient's family may also require counselling.

DISCHARGE FROM CRITICAL CARE

Leaving CCU environment can be upsetting for a patient, even if they have had a short stay. They may no longer require monitoring in the same way, and this may lead to anxiety, and a feeling that they have been "abandoned"; or that there will be no one to notice if "something goes wrong". Relatives may also be unduly concerned about the change in environment, and ward staff may be concerned about their ability to care for the patient.

Many hospitals have now adopted a critical care outreach approach to caring for these patients. This is designed to:

1. support the patient on the ward;
2. support the ward staff in caring for these patients;
3. monitor the patient for complications, and to ensure that ward staff are supported in dealing with them;
4. ensure that the patient is readmitted to ITU as soon as possible if required.

Outreach services develop according to a particular hospital's need, and can range from the provision of a telephone advice line, to a type of "crash team". In many situations, the team will be multi-disciplinary, including doctors, nurses and physiotherapists.

KEY POINTS

- Vascular surgery patients usually need to spend some time in a critical care environment. This may be due to concurrent medical problems, the methods of pain relief employed, the occurrence of complications or the nature of surgery performed.
- The monitoring of the patient post-operatively will always consist of basic physiological measurements, supplemented by observations related specifically to the type of surgery undergone. Equipment being used to support the patient (e.g. ventilators, etc.) should also be monitored to prevent malfunction. *Prevention of complications is better than a cure.*
- A CCU utilises a higher nursing–patient ratio. There is access to additional therapies for providing support to failing organs.
- Complications may require an urgent return to theatre, or a transfer to a higher level of care. *Early detection is essential.* Regular observations and

attention to detail in the care of these patients are the keys to a successful outcome.
- Even patients who have spent only a short period of time in CCU may require support from the outreach staff after discharge.
- Patients who have spent a prolonged period of time in CCU may require access to specialist follow-up or rehabilitative services.

FURTHER READING

Comprehensive Critical Care DoH (2000).

Grant I & Singer M (eds) (1999) *ABC of Intensive Care*. BMJ books.

Griffiths RD & Jones C (2002) *Intensive Care Aftercare*. Butterworth Heinmann.

McConachie I (ed.) (2002) *Anaesthesia for the High Risk Patient*. GMM.

Ridley S, Smith G & Batchelor A (eds) (2003) *Core Cases in Critical Care*. GMM.

Smith G (2000) Alert: *A Multiprofessional Course in Care of the Acutely Ill Patient*. University of Portsmouth/Intensive Care Society.

The Nursing Contribution to the Provision of Comprehensive Critical Care for Adults DoH (2001).

TRAINING AND PRACTICE ISSUES

6.1 THE ROLE OF THE VASCULAR NURSE SPECIALIST

L. Thompson

Caring for patients with vascular disease is a complex and challenging area of care for all involved. The need for the provision of specialist nursing input to meet the requirements of vascular patients is now widely recognised. The role of the vascular nurse specialist can be divided into separate areas, all of equal importance. The areas I will be discussing can be divided into three sections as follows: *education, advice and support, research and development.*

EDUCATION

Education of patients and their relatives: The main emphasis being the provision of health education using research-based evidence. It is the role of the vascular nurse to assist patients to make lifestyle changes from the earliest stages of the disease. Once an initial assessment has been made and risk factors identified, it is necessary to plan, implement and evaluate appropriate, realistic interventions. In the case of patients with vascular disease this usually involves a number of different aspects of lifestyle including smoking cessation, good control of blood pressure and diabetes, advice on diet, cholesterol and exercise, and advice on good food care.

Education of staff: It is also the role of the vascular nurse to ensure the educational needs of nursing staff and other members of the multi-disciplinary team are met, by the provision of educational training and the teaching of clinical skills. It is important to identify training needs and plan regular training sessions to meet these requirements.

ADVICE AND SUPPORT

The second area to consider is that of advice and support in both the pre- and post-operative phase. It is vital that the patient has enough knowledge and information about proposed treatment to make an informed decision about their care. By discussing information regarding disease and treatment options, and providing written information about any proposed surgery, the vascular nurse specialist can ensure if patients are empowered to make an informed choice about their care.

By providing a contact service for the patients at this time, any worries or concerns can be addressed at any time.

It is also important to act as a resource to other health care professionals by again providing advice and support to enable them to care for patients with both competence and confidence.

RESEARCH AND DEVELOPMENT

For every vascular nurse specialist it is vital that research-based practice is both implemented and promoted.

It is also important to demonstrate commitment to the development of one's own research skills, and to disseminate current research ideas for further investigation.

SUMMARY OF THE ROLE OF THE VASCULAR NURSE SPECIALIST

- To provide expert vascular nursing advice, support and education to patients, carers, nursing staff and members of the multi-disciplinary team.
- To be actively involved in the pre- and post-operative care of patients/ relatives.
- To promote vascular disease awareness and its prevention.
- To participate in the assessment of patient and carer needs, and evaluate programmes of care.
- To assist in compiling reports, and participate in research projects and audit.

REFERENCE

Vascular Disease, Nursing and Management, Shelagh Murray, Whurr Publishers, London and Philadelphia.

6.2   TRAINING FOR VASCULAR NURSES

S. Dorgan

The growth of vascular nursing as a recognised specialist area is reflected in the opportunities to undertake courses at various centres in the UK. These courses have arisen over the last decade and there are opportunities for vascular nurses to study at two centres in London and one in Liverpool. By successfully completing a course, nurses can obtain 30–40 credits at Level 2 or 3, depending on the chosen course.

The courses are aimed at health care professionals working with people with vascular disease, in either acute or community clinical settings. It is hoped that such study will equip nurses with the appropriate skills and knowledge to ensure high quality and evidence-based care for patients with vascular disorders.

Course content varies. Topics covered include health promotion, anatomy and physiology, ethical and professional issues, patient management and rehabilitation.

Listed below are contact details for each of the three centres.

Vascular nursing (formerly ENB U06) at the Faculty of Health and Social Care Sciences – Kingston University – St George's Hospital Medical School.

Further information:
Denise Forte Tel: 020 8547 8728

Applications to:
Post Registration Admissions Office
Faculty of Health and Social Care Sciences
St George's Hospital Medical School
Cranmer Terrace
London SW17 0RE

Vascular nursing (formerly ENB A85 Module) at the Centre for Research and Implementation of Clinical Practice – Wolfson Institute of Health Sciences, London.

Enquiries and application forms:
Rene White
Course Administrator
Faculty of Health and Human Sciences
Thames Valley University
32–38 Uxbridge Road
London W5 2BS

Vascular nursing course (HEA 354, formerly ENB U06) at the School of Health Studies – University Hospital Aintree Site, Liverpool.

Course Co-ordinator Jim Gorman
Tel: 0151 529 3718 or gormanj@edgehill.ac.uk

Application forms available from Vicki Hall
Tel: 0151 529 3084 or hallv@edgehill.ac.uk

6.3 INTEGRATED CARE PATHWAYS

S. Dorgan

INTRODUCTION

Structured care relates to strategies for controlling both the cost and quality of clinical interventions, and incorporates innovations like case management, care pathways, managed care and care packages. The impetus for these developments came from cost-orientated schemes to standardise health care within the USA. Initiatives in the National Health Services (NHS) focusing on financial (Department of Health & Social Services [DHSS], 1991) and subsequently clinical (Department of Health [DoH], 1993) effectiveness have culminated in a national clinical governance framework (DoH, 1998) whereby individual health care trusts are charged with ensuring the quality of their care.

Trusts are expected to:

- audit their care;
- demonstrate its evidence base;
- monitor its outcomes;
- deal quickly with any areas of poor practice. Consequently, structured care schemes, with their emphasis on defining and controlling the processes behind care delivery are in the forefront of contemporary clinical developments (Laxade & Hale, 1995).

DEFINITION OF INTEGRATED CARE PATHWAYS

The care pathway is a set of guidelines for providing care to patients with specific medical conditions. It incorporates interventions and treatments along with the expected intermediate goals and clinical outcomes. The clinical pathway is defined by diagnosis or by condition.

They seek to improve quality care by co-ordinating the timing of specific interventions and allocating them to the most appropriate health care professional (Hale, 1995).

With a care pathway, the patients' health care needs are tracked across the entire continuum of care, from pre-admission through hospitalisation to outpatient and clinical care. The essential elements of a clinical pathway are a timeline and a list of problems, interventions and outcomes. Deviations from the pathway interventions and outcomes are coded as variances.

Purpose

Designed by the multi-disciplinary team (MDT), the purpose of a care pathway is to:

- Improve the quality of care provided to patients.
- Minimise delays in treatments.
- Maximise the use of all available resources.
- Reduce length of stay in hospital.
- Reduce cost per episode of care.

It is a communication tool that all disciplines can use to facilitate the co-ordination of patient care.

POTENTIAL BENEFITS AND CRITICISMS OF INTEGRATED CARE PATHWAYS

Integrated care pathways (ICPs) provide a specific sequence of events or treatments for hospitalised and community-based patients. The listed multi-disciplinary interventions and actions for specific surgical interventions (e.g. carotid endarterectomy) or medical conditions (e.g. stroke) are within a designated time frame (Hoxie, 1996; Allen, 1997). ICPs have many advantages as listed in Table 6.3.1. Criticism of pathways centres on the issue of standardising care in terms of the points are highlighted in Table 6.3.2.

Table 6.3.1: Potential benefits of ICPs

- Standardising the core expectations of clinical input for particular procedures
- Minimising repetition of activity and hence reducing paperwork
- Improving multi-disciplinary communication
- Enhancing client understanding of their progress and practitioner accountability
- Improving discharge information and arrangements
- Providing guidance and direction to newly appointed practitioners
- Identifying interventions that frequently prove to be problematic

Source: Nelson, 1995.

Table 6.3.2: Criticisms of ICPs

- Their impact on individual autonomy and clinical decision-making
- The difficulties in securing agreement from the variety of professions on:
  - which interventions should be included in each pathway
  - who has responsibility for their completion

Source: Nelson, 1995.

Categories

Care pathways are usually divided into eight categories, although this will vary according to individual organisations who develop them (Table 6.3.3). The categories usually include:

- tests,
- treatments,
- consultations,
- diet,
- medications,
- activity,
- teaching,
- discharge planning.

Variances

Certain complex health care problems require deviations from the core clinical pathway format for patients with special needs. These situations are documented on a variance form, which may be attached to the core clinical pathway. This is a related document to be used concurrently with a clinical pathway, usually as an attachment. Therefore a variance is a deviation from the pathway. Pathways should be reviewed on a daily basis to ensure variance identification. The MDT should then take action to get the patient back on tack. There are four types of variance:

- patient,
- caregiver,
- system,
- community.

Variances can be positive (where the patient recovers quicker than the anticipated recovery time), negative (where the patient takes longer than expected to recover), avoidable and unavoidable.

Table 6.3.3: ICP for varicose veins

Categories	Date: Pre-admission	Sign	Date: Day of surgery		Sign	Post-operative	Sign	Date: Discharge day (surgery + [1])	Sign
			Pre-operative						
Desired outcomes	• Patient verbalises understanding of reasons for surgery, knowledge of the procedure, and is prepared for forthcoming admission.		• Patient verbalises understanding of reasons for varicose vein surgery, the risks involved and is prepared for surgery.			• Patient is haemo-dynamically stable, pain is controlled.		• Uneventful recovery from treatment allowing patient to safely be discharged home.	
Tests	• *Bloods:* FBC, U+E's, clotting, glucose (if diabetic), • Duplex scan, Vital signs, ECG and CXR (if required).		Ensure have: • Blood results • Scans (duplex/ECG/X-ray).						
Teaching	• Pre-operative teaching handout on varicose veins. • Discuss care pathway. • Discharge advice leaflet.		• Check patients understanding of: – nurse call system – post-operative: O$_2$, IVI, pain, dressings.			• Deep breathing exercises. • Leg exercises.		• Reiterate discharge information. • If surgery has involved short saphenous vein, ensure prolene stitches are removed in 10/7.	

(continued)

Table 6.3.3: (Continued)

Categories	Date: Pre-admission	Sign	Date: Day of surgery Pre-operative	Sign	Post-operative	Sign	Date: Discharge day (surgery + [1])	Sign
Medication	• Review medication: – where patient takes stock drugs advise to leave at home – for non-stock drugs advise to bring along on admission day.		• Ensure all medication taken – cardiac/ epileptic drugs, etc. • Commence sliding scale insulin, if required. • Give clexane s/c 20 mg.		• Restart medication when patient able to tolerate diet/fluid.		• Return patients own medication. • Give patient any prescribed medication to take home and explain dosage, side effects.	
Diet	• Establish if special diet is required. • Advise re: pre-operative fasting.		• Ensure patient is fasted 4/6 h prior to surgery. If fasted >12 h, inform medics.		• Offer patient diet/ fluids when patient able to tolerate.			
Interventions	• Complete demographic details. • Complete medical history. • Measure and order TED stockings. • Obtain informed consent.		• Ensure surgeon marks legs. • Apply TED stocking to non-surgical leg prior to theatre.		• Record BP, P, T, Sat 1 hourly, reduce as patients health dictates. • Ensure urine passed in 12 h. • Check wound.		• Check wound prior to discharge, observing for swelling. • Advise patient to wear stockings for 2/52.	

Discharge planning	• Document length of stay. • Discuss transport requirements.	• Clarify discharge/GP letter. • Book transport for following day if required.	• Complete district nurse referral. • Book outpatient appointment for 6 weeks.	• Ensure OPA booked 6/52. • Ensure district nurse booked. • Give discharge info leaflet. • Book OPA transport if required.
Completion	Nurse sign: _____ Print name: _____ Date: _____	Date: _____ Nurse sign: _____ Print name: _____ am: _____ pm: _____	Date: _____ Nurse sign: _____ Print name: _____ am: _____ pm: _____	Nurse sign: _____ Print name: _____ Date: _____

FBC: full blood count; U+E: urea and electrolytes; ECG: electrocardiogram; CXR: chest X-ray; IVI: intravenous injection; GP: general practitioner; BP: blood pressure; P: pulse rate TED: thrombo embolism deterrent; OPA: outpatient appointment.

QUALITY CONTROL

Clinical pathways that incorporate quality improvement indices are valuable to the clinician and the health care organisation. The quality improvement process is a structured series of steps designed to plan, evaluate and propose changes for health care activities. Improvement in health care activities would be necessary when: multi-variances occur; patients do not achieve expected outcomes; referrals are not seen within a specified time period; length of stay is extended and patient/family education is not documented within a specified time period. Indicators are generally used by the institution quality control team and are not a permanent part of the chart, but may be attached to the pathway to ensure assessment by the health care team.

Advantages of care pathways

For the patient
- Stresses the continuity of patient care and the services rendered.
- Collaboration between patients and professional disciplines is encouraged. This is said to have a positive impact on the quality of patient care.

For the clinician
- Setting out what clinicians do.
- Seeing if we are doing the same thing.
- Agreeing with the same things.
- Comparing it to evidence base.

For the trust
- Patient care will be provided in a fiscally responsible length of stay.
- As the care pathway specifies the resources required, duplication of services is reduced.
- Improvements in care can be achieved by constantly ensuring that feedback is used to rectify the shortcomings identified.
- Efficient, effective and evidence-based care.
- It is a risk management tool.

THE KEY TO SUCCESS

The key ingredients for successful introduction of care pathways include sustained leadership, and provision of an infrastructure to complete the necessary research, including high-quality clinical audit staff.

Whilst the benefits of care pathways are widely known and documented, the scheme does not offer a quick-fix solution, and it is highly unlikely that a pathway which works in one organisation can be acquired and used successfully in another. It may be the same condition and outcome with identical disciplines involved, but it will always be somebody else's pathway. Each organisation needs to invent its own pathway if they are to believe in it.

How to implement integrated care pathways

- Identify patient group for ICP.
- Identify MDT involved with this patient group, contact one member from each discipline to sit on steering group.
- Discuss about the project with the audit team and involve from the outset.
- Initial meeting is to discuss ICP development.
- Look at the current practice, identify areas that require improvement and areas of best practice.
- Undertake comprehensive literature review.
- Formulate draft ICP document.
- Follow a patient through the system using the pathway.
- Identify any changes to the ICP.
- Implement full education and training package for all involved ICP users.
- Agree set date for pilot study and time span.
- Launch pilot ICP.
- Audit pilot ICP.
- Presentation of pilot ICP findings.
- Update any ICP document changes.
- Implement ICP.
- Ongoing monitoring will be required and changes made according to new evidence-based practice and guidelines.

REFERENCES

Allen CV (1997) *Nursing Process in Collaborative Practice*, 2nd Edition. Appelton & Lange, Stamford CT.

Department of Health and Social Services Inspectorate (1991) *Care Management and Assessment – Practitioners' Guide and Managers' Guide*. HMSO, London.

Department of Health (1993) *Hospital Doctors' Training for the Future. Report of the Working Group on Specialist Medical Training (the Calman Report)*. DoH, London.

Department of Health (1998) *A First Class Service: Quality in the New NHS*. HMSO, London.

Hale C (1995) Case management and managed care. *Nurs Stand* 9(19): 33–35.

Hoxie LO (1996) Outcomes, measurements and clinical pathways. *J Prosth Orthot* 8(3): 93–95.

Laxade S & Hale C (1995) Managed care 1: an opportunity for nursing. *Br J Nurs* 4(5): 290–294.

Nelson S (1995) Following pathways in pursuit of excellence. *Int J Health Care Quality Assurance* 8(7): 19–22.

6.4 CLINICAL GOVERNANCE

V. Skinner

Definition

Governance is the stewardship of the valuable resources (time, money, equipment, and skills) for which someone has directly or indirectly been given the responsibility.

CLINICAL GOVERNANCE

"Clinical Governance is the framework through which National Health Services (NHS) organisations are accountable for continually improving the quality of their services and safeguarding high standards of care by creating an environment in which excellence in clinical care will flourish" (Scally & Donaldson, 1998).

- Clinical Governance became the vehicle for delivering quality improvements and assuring the quality of care expected by the document "A First Class Service: Quality in the New NHS" (1998).
- Clinical Governance (quality assurance) became the responsibility of every chief executive of an NHS Trust.
- Clinical Governance seeks to change the culture of the NHS and making quality of service an integral part of everyday life for NHS staff.

The Clinical Governance process

Clinical Governance requires a multi-professional approach to care:

- care standards,
- audit,
- improvements based on research or other documented evidence.

This multi-profession team can be the Directorate Management Team or a completely separate body but it must have the authority to action change and report to the Trust Board and/or its Clinical Governance Committee.

The "team" will lead, guide, support and report on all Clinical Governance issues within the directorate. The "team" will be expected to use the National Guide to facilitate Clinical Governance, e.g.:

1. Review the service provided.
2. Agree health care improvements.
3. Implement quality improvements.
4. Demonstrate that changes have taken place, and the degree of effect those changes have had on patients, service and staff.

The Commission for Health Improvement (CHI) review NHS Trust's Clinical Governance using seven pre-designated areas:

1. Patient involvement.
2. Patient experience.
3. Staffing and staff management.
4. Training and continuous professional development.
5. Clinical risk management.
6. Clinical audit.
7. Research and effectiveness.

Each of these areas are detailed as follows.

Patient involvement

There are no set guidelines for how you should involve patients, their relatives and/or the general public. However, it must be borne in mind that the reason for involving patients and the public in Clinical Governance is to get their views on how the service could be improved to benefit both themselves and the service providers.

Therefore patients need to have a greater understanding of what the trusts are attempting to do and the targets they have to meet. The people who would be involved will need to access staff and patients, and gain the respect and confidence of both.

Questions that might help you to involve patients

- Is there a policy stating how the users are to be selected/interviewed/reimbursed for out of pocket expenses?
- How are patients informed of changes within the services now?
- How are patients involved in the planning and provision of services?
- How patients involved in clinical audit and clinical risk activities?
- How would patients be involved in the selection and monitoring of research projects?

Patient's and relatives experiences

Patient's views are extremely valuable if used to their full potential. Most NHS staff over the past 10 years has sought the views of their patients via patient satisfaction surveys, which have had varying degrees of success.

What is needed is an objective picture of the life of a patient during their stay in hospital and their journey before and after the period of hospitalisation. Suggestions for obtaining the views of patients, their relatives and visitors are as follows:

- *Patient's diary*: To be kept by the patient from arrival in the outpatient clinic, through the period of hospitalisation, discharge and community follow-up. Positive, as well as negative things, should be recorded in the diary:
  - What went well for the patient?
  - What did they feel could have been done better?
  - Did they always get what was promised?
  - How long did they have to wait before getting the information or equipment once they had made the request?
  - How were the patients kept informed of the tests done and the subsequent results?
  - How were they informed of the diagnosis and were they given any options for the treatments?
- *Patient interviews/stories*: Whereby staff trained in interviewing techniques could interview patients immediately following discharge either from the service or following discharge from hospital.
- *Patient forums*: Held for patients or those held specifically for relatives and carers can give a lot of valuable information about the service and their expectations.
- *Patient complaints*: "Organisations with a Memory" demonstrates how organisations can learn from examples of poor practice to ensure that the same mistakes are not made over and over again.
- *Casenote reviews*: Reading of patient notes following discharge gives a full picture of the patient's clinical experience, especially where the notes contain the information from each health professional who have delivered treatment.
- *CHI reviews*: When the commission visits an NHS organisation, the team hold several meetings to get the views of their users and the feedback from these meetings could be very useful to the trust.

Staffing and staff management

- Staffing and the value of staff are important for the running of large organisations.

- Staff must have the relevant qualifications for the post to which they are appointed and have a valid licence to practise.
- Staff needs to ensure that they have specialised training in order to carry out "specialist" duties, this will include training in various pieces of equipment until they are sure they understand how it works, how to monitor its functions and what records should be kept regarding its use.
- Where staff do not understand what is being asked of them, they should report this to the person in charge of the ward/department.
- Appropriate staffing levels vary dependent on the dependency levels of their patients, the number of patients, how seriously ill they are now and is that expected to deteriorate during the shift and the type of care being delivered.

Training and continuous professional development

Staff require time and support to undertake personal and professional development in order to provide the highest standards of care for patients, to include:

- annual appraisal of each member of staff with an action plan for development;
- annual assessment of training needs with an action plan to meet those needs;
- regular review of the portfolio by the individual member of staff with or without support from their clinical supervisor, line manager or trainer.

Clinical risk management

- Clinical and non-clinical risk management is linked together and forms an essential part of Clinical Governance.
- Clinical risk assessments are undertaken to prevent the re-occurrence of an incident and not to find a person to blame, there is also a responsibility to ensure that prevention is trust wide and not just directorate wide.
- Every incident, be it clinical incident, security incident, accident or any near misses, needs to be followed up independently to assess potential risk for the trust.
- A simple but mandatory system for the reporting of incidents which needs to include "a no blame culture" in order for staff to report near misses.
- A system for grading of the incidents.
- Communications between clinical audit and the various Clinical Governance Committees and the risk manager in order that action plans can be easily developed to prevent the repetition of incidents.
- Clinical audit can undertake audit of clinical practices or clinical processes in order to determine the root of a problem or incident.

- Identification of "trends", which need to be investigated furthering order to identify where the problem arises.
- Serious incidents require the facilitation of a Critical Incident Panel to identify avoidable factors and put in place actions to prevent re-occurrence.

Clinical audit

- Is a statutory requirement for medical staff and over the last 6 years has been an expected activity for all other clinical staff.
- It is normally a multi-professional team activity with a representative from each profession caring for a specific group of patients which should also include a patient or member of the public.
- Each audit project should have a team of professionals plus a member of the public who will review the standards to be audited, set the audit tool, undertake the audit, write the report and set the action plan.
- Standards are reviewed in the light of National Institute for Clinical Excellence (NICE) Guidelines, National Service Framework standards and any research that has been undertaken.
- National Enquiries which review all deaths occurring in hospitals produce reports of their findings with particular reference to avoidable factors. These indicators should also be implemented with a view to audit to determine the improvement in practice.
- Education of staff in clinical audit techniques and development of tools/databases/critical appraisal of research findings and development of action plans is undertaken by clinical audit departments.
- British Standards Institute for BS EN ISO 2000, National External Auditors are independent auditors:
  - e.g. Health Service Quality (formally Kings Fund Organisational Audit), CHI and the Audit Commission.

Research and effectiveness

Research is the systematic search for new knowledge that will have an effect on patients. In the last decade there has been much controversy and several legal cases on the conduct of researchers undertaking Health Service Research. Therefore, it is transpired that the Department of Health produced a comprehensive Research Governance Framework for Health and Social Care 2001.

This document:

- Sets standards.
- Defines mechanisms to deliver the standards.
- Describes monitoring and assessment by the Department of Health.

- Improves research quality and safeguards the public by:
  – enhancing ethical and scientific quality,
  – promoting good practice,
  – reducing adverse incidents and ensuring lessons are learnt,
  – prevents poor performance and misconduct.

This document is for all staff working in Health and Social Care, no matter how senior or how junior in both primary and secondary care.

The main principles

The main principles are as follows:

- Has the researcher the skills to undertake the research?
- Discussion of the proposal with the research manager or co-ordinator.
- Obtain an academic and clinical supervisor.
- Obtain two independent review reports on the methodology.
- Identify the sponsor.
- Ensure that all the costs are accounted for and that funding is approved.
- All respondent information is in a format that they can read and understand.
- Ethical approval from the appropriate body has been sought and received.
- A system is in place to record and report all adverse incidents.
- Ensure that if amendments are made to the protocol for whatever reason the following bodies are informed before the new protocol is used:
  – Research manager
  – Funding body
  – Ethics committee
  – Sponsor
  – Supervisor

Data for each research project must be kept for as long as is necessary for anyone to query the findings following publication or as long as the Trust Policy states.

CONSENT

Informed consent to participate in research should be given freely when the person to be involved has read and understood what will be expected of them.

It should be given by the person to be involved in the research but this may depend on the study, the ethical committee and/or others involved in the research approval.

ETHICS GOVERNANCE

Ethical Committees have their own Governance document, which is available from the Department of Health web site.

RECOMMENDED READING

A First Class Service: Quality in the New NHS 1998.
Ethics Governance Framework 2002.
Implementing Clinical Governance – Progress so far 2003. Professor A Halligen.
Research Governance Framework for Health and Social Care 2001.
Scally G & Donaldson LM (1998) "Clinical Governance and the drive for quality improvement in the "New NHS" in England". *Br Med J* 317: 61–65.
The NHS Plan: Quality in the New NHS 1998.

FURTHER INFORMATION

www.doh.gov.uk
www.doh.gov.uk/research
www.corec.gov.uk
www.audit-commission.gov.uk
www.nice.org.uk

USEFUL CONTACTS

1. The Patients Association   www.patients-association.com/
2. Age Concern   www.ageconcern.org.uk/
3. British Heart Foundation   www.bhf.org.uk
4. Diabetes UK   www.diabetes.org.uk
5. MIND Mental Health Charity   www.mind.org.uk
6. Cystic Fibrosis   www.iacfa.org
                                  www.cff.org

7. Epilepsy Association   www.epilepsy.org.uk

6.5   AUDIT

F. Serracino-Inglott

What is Audit?

Audit is the process by which medical, nursing and paramedical staff assess their practice with a view towards improving their standards. Audit can be carried out at various levels of patient care. Medical audit involves the assessment of the medical care provided by the medical profession to the patient by peer review. An example of this would be morbidity and mortality meetings. Clinical audit has a much broader remit, encompassing the multi-disciplinary assessment of the effects of health care by all health professionals on the patient as a whole.

Medical audit became formalised in the UK following the publication of the white paper *Working for Patients* in 1989. This defined *medical audit* as *the systematic critical analysis of quality of medical care including the procedures used for diagnosis and treatment, the use of resources and the resulting outcome and quality of life for the patient.* In 1993 the National Health Services (NHS) Management Executive integrated medical, nursing and therapy audit programmes coining the term *clinical audit*. This was defined as *the systematic critical analysis of the quality of health care, including the procedures used for diagnosis treatment and care, the use of resources and the resulting outcome and quality of life for patients,* to embrace the work of all health professionals. When *Clinical Governance* was introduced in 1997, one of its integral elements was clinical audit; the other elements being education, clinical effectiveness, risk management, research and development, and openness. The most up to date definition of clinical audit has recently been published by the National Institute for Clinical Excellence (NICE) and is given below:

> Clinical audit is a quality improvement process that seeks to improve patient care and outcomes through systematic review of care against explicit criteria and the implementation of change. Aspects of the structure, processes and outcomes of care are selected, and systematically evaluated against explicit criteria. Where indicated, changes are implemented at an individual, team or service level and further monitoring is used to confirm improvement in health care delivery.

THE AUDIT CYCLE

The audit cycle is based on three main questions:

1. What should be happening?
2. What is actually happening?
3. What changes should be implemented for the answer to question 2 to be closer to that for question 1?

And on implementing the answer to question 3. This will contribute towards:

- Improving patient care.
- Increasing professionalism.
- More efficient use of resources.
- Better accountability.
- Learning.

Figure 6.5.1 depicts the audit cycle, each step of which will be discussed in more detail later in the text. The cycle is repeated until one's results are as close as possible to the set criteria and standards.

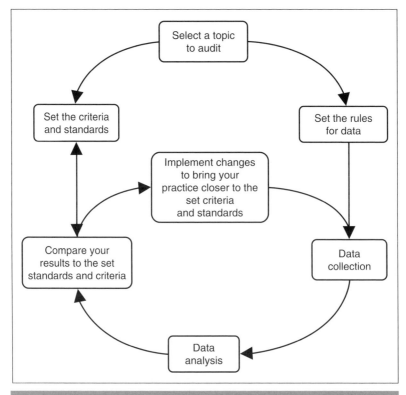

Fig. 6.5.1: The audit cycle.

What to audit?

When deciding what to audit you should choose a subject that you consider to have clinical importance or significance. Think through exactly what you want your audit to be about and what you want it to achieve. You then need to identify a measurable item that can be used to assess it. For example, it is important that patients with peripheral vascular disease are started on an antiplatelet agent, such as aspirin or clopidogrel. Therefore, you can choose to measure the percentage of patients with intermittent claudication who leave the vascular clinic on an antiplatelet agent. Sources for clinically important audit topics may be found by looking up patient complaints and subjects published by the NICE. You could, e.g. look into whether the new recommendations for preoperative investigations recently published by NICE being adhered to.

All audits should contain criteria that are evidence based. If this is absent further research into this area is required. Although both research and audit may involve measuring patient outcomes, the purpose of each is different. In research one uses the results to arrive to conclusions on what really works or is more effective. This usually involves comparing different procedures thought to have relatively similar outcomes. On the other hand, clinical audit monitors outcomes to see if they achieve pre-determined expectations. To put it in simpler terms, *research* asks the question *what is best clinical practice?* whilst *clinical audit* asks *is best clinical practice being practiced?* Prior to embarking on an audit project you then need to be able to explain to others how your chosen audit is based on solid research as well as how it will contribute to the quality and efficacy of patient care.

SETTING THE CRITERIA AND STANDARDS

Setting the standards describes the level of care expected for any particular criterion. For example, it is important that the criteria you choose are those:

- Which are essential rather than optional – e.g. one would expect that all patients with intermittent claudication should be on an antiplatelet agent unless they have a bleeding diathesis.
- For which sound research evidence exists, e.g. all claudicants should be advised to embark on an exercise programme.
- Which can be easily audited using patient records, e.g. *claudicants should have their ankle brachial pressure index checked yearly* is difficult to measure, while *how many claudicants have had their ankle brachial pressure checked last year?* is more practical.
- Which are realistic practices given the capacity of a facility in terms of staff and resources – in some specialities *National Service Frameworks* lay out the standards to be expected.

DATA COLLECTION

Data for audit purposes can be collected *retrospectively* or *prospectively*. *Retrospective collection* means that the data is collected from patient records or from sources, such as operation theatre books. The records may be in paper form, or in electronic form. It is important that a systematic approach is used to search these sources to avoid either missing or double-counting cases. In all cases, it is also important to ensure that there is suitable *anonymisation* of data, i.e. there is no information which can enable the patient to be identified, in order to preserve patient confidentiality. When the number of cases is too large for all the patient records to be reviewed, then a representative sample may be selected, however, this must be done with caution. For example, if one needs to find out the ratio of above-knee to below-knee amputations, one does not need to go through all the patient records but one can select a sample of around 50 patients at random. The main disadvantage of retrospective data collection is that not all the information required may be found in the patient records. This disadvantage does not exist with prospective data collection.

Prospective data collection means that the data pertaining to the event is collected as it happens rather than at a later date. An example of this is the recording of the POSSUM scale (Physiological and Operative Severity Score for the enUmeration of Mortality and morbidity) where the form is filled in during the pre-operative assessment, right after the surgical procedure, and at discharge. The main disadvantage of prospective data collection is the time for the final data to be available is dependent on the length of the study period.

COMPARING YOUR PRACTICE WITH THE STANDARD PRACTICE

The results obtained from the data collection process are compared to the previously defined standard practice. It is important to make sure that the same units of measurement are used for comparison.

MODIFYING YOUR PRACTICE

After identifying areas for improvement, an action plan should be draughted. For example, if not enough patients with intermittent claudication are being released on antiplatelet medication, actions to be taken could include sending a reminder to the involved clinicians to do so, visual reminders, such as posters in the clinic, and the addition of a reminder to the clinic letter template. Actually making the proposed changes is the most difficult part of the audit cycle. Changes are more likely to succeed if they are practical and if the staff who need to implement the change are all involved in the modifying process.

CLOSING THE LOOP

The audit should be repeated to make sure that the modifications instituted have made your practice more similar to the set criteria. If this is not the case, further modifications should be instituted and the audit cycle repeated. This is probably the most important part of the audit cycle since it confirms that your changes have had an effect on improving clinical outcome.

NATIONAL VASCULAR DATABASE AND V-POSSUM

The National Vascular Database is kept by the Vascular Surgical Society of Great Britain and Ireland. Data relating to all index vascular operations (carotid endarterectomy, abdominal aortic aneurysm repair and infra-inguinal bypass) are submitted by more than 200 surgeons from various centres. This database now contains around 6000 index procedures that are available for analysis. The advantage of having such a large data set is that it allows risk models to be constructed. Operative mortality and morbidity will vary between vascular teams because of reasons other than the team's performance. These include case-mix, co-morbid disease and type of presentation. Risk models have the potential to compensate for these factors and therefore allow a better means of auditing a surgeon's performance.

POSSUM stands for Physiological and Operative Severity Score for the enUmeration of Mortality and morbidity. It was developed by *Copeland and co-workers* and has since been applied to a number of surgical procedures. POSSUM aims to adjust the risk of a surgical procedure based on the patient's physiological condition and therefore allow a more accurate comparison of a team's performance. Twelve physiological (including age, systolic blood pressure and heart rate) and six operative (including operative blood loss and peritoneal contamination) parameters are measured. Each of these 18 factors are weighted and used in a formula to calculate the predicted mortality and morbidity. *Prytherch and colleagues* modified the original POSSUM formula for use in elective vascular surgery. When applied to Vascular surgery it carries the V-prefix. With the increasing emphasis on informed consent such a scoring system is particularly useful in giving individual patient's information regarding the morbidity and mortality of a procedure that are specific to their overall state of health. For example, the mortality following elective abdominal aortic aneurysm repair for an 80-year-old patient with heart failure and high blood pressure is going to be much higher than that of a 65-year-old patient with no co-morbidity.

Both the National Vascular Database and V-POSSUM allow the comparison of like with like. This is of paramount importance if clinical audit is to achieve its goal of improving the quality of health care.

FURTHER READING

All web sites accessed 19/01/2004.

Ashley S, Riddler B & Kinsman R (2002) *National Vascular Database Report*. Dendrite Clinical Systems Ltd., Bull Inn Courtyard, 59A Bell Street, Henley-on-Thames, Oxfordshire, RG9 2BA. Available from http://www.vssgbi.org/Docs/NVD2002.pdf

North Bristol NHS Trust (2002) Clinical Audit Department, *What is Audit?* Available from: http://www.northbristol.nhs.uk/depts/ClinicalGovernance/ClinicalAudit/display_page.asp?id=42

Harris M (2003). *Study Guide – Clinical Audit*. Available from: http://www.mharris.eurobell.co.uk/contents.htm

Hine D & Rawlins M (2002) *Principles for Best Practice in Clinical Audit*. Radcliffe Medical Press Ltd. Available from http://www.nelh.nhs.uk/BestPracticeClinicalAudit.pdf

Kennedy I (2001) Learning from Bristol. The report of the public inquiry into children's heart surgery at the Bristol Royal Infirmary 1984–1995 Chapter 18. *Medical and Clinical Audit*. London: The Stationery Office. Available from: http://www.bristol-inquiry.org.uk/final%5Freport/annex_a/chapter_18_.htm

Smith J & Tekkis P Vascular-POSSUM Scoring. Available from: http://www.riskprediction.org.uk/vasc-index.php

The Cochrane Library. Update Software Ltd, Summertown Pavilion, Middle Way, OXFORD OX2 7LG, UK. Available from: www.update-software.com/cochrane/

Thomas K & Emberton M (2002) *Modern Surgical Audit*. Available from: http://www.medicinepublishing.com/2_1.htm

6.6 USEFUL ADDRESSES

Action on Smoking & Health (ASH)
16 Fitzharding Street
London
W1H 9LP
Tel: 0171 224 0743
Fax: 0171 224 0471

Amputee Medical Rehabilitation Society
The Royal College of Physicians
St Andrews Place
London
NW1

British Diabetic Association
10 Queen Anne Street
London
W1M 0BP
Tel: 0171 323 1531
Fax: 0171 637 3644
Help line: 0171 636 6112

British Heart Foundation
14 Fitzhardinge Street
London
W1H 4DH
Tel: 0171 935 0185
Heart line: 0990 200 656

British Vascular Foundation
Griffin House
West Street
Woking
Surrey
GU21 1EB
Tel: 01483 726511
Fax: 01483 726522

Lymphoedema Support Network
St Lukes Crypt
Sydney Street
London
SW3 6NH
Tel: 0171 351 4480
Fax: 0171 349 9809

Raynaud's and Scleroderma Association
112 Crewe Road
Alsagar
Cheshire
ST7 2JA
Tel: 01270 872776
Fax: 01270 883556

The Stroke Association
Stroke House
Whitecross Street
London
EC1Y 8JJ
Tel: 0171 490 7999

Vascular Surgical Society of Great Britain & Ireland
Royal College of Surgeons
35–43 Lincolns Inn Fields
London
WC2A 3PN
Tel: 020 7973 0306
Fax: 020 7430 9235

INDEX

DATE DUE

Demco, Inc. 38-293